THE FACE
OF THE
FUTURE

LOOK NATURAL, NOT PLASTIC:
A LESS-INVASIVE APPROACH
TO ENHANCE YOUR BEAUTY
AND REVERSE FACIAL AGING

ANDREW A. JACONO, MD, FACS

Addicus Books
Omaha, Nebraska

An Addicus Nonfiction Book

ISBN 978-1-936374-87-8
Cover design by Gary Wong, interior design by Jack Kusler
Illustrations by William M. Winn, M.S.
Cover photo by William Hereford
This book is not intended to serve as a substitute for a physician, nor is it the author's intent to give medical advice contrary to that of an attending physician.

Library of Congress Cataloging-in-Publication Data

Jacono, Andrew A., 1970-
   Face of the future : look natural not plastic : a less-invasive approach to enhance your beauty and reverse facial aging / Andrew A. Jacono.
       p. cm.
   Includes bibliographical references and index.
   ISBN 978-1-936374-87-8 (alk. paper)
1. Face--Surgery--Popular works. 2.   Surgery, Plastic--Popular works. 3.   Beauty, Personal--Popular works. 4.   Skin--Care and hygiene--Popular works.   I. Title.
   RD523.J35 2012
   617.5'20592--dc23

                                                  2012021553

Addicus Books, Inc.
P.O. Box 45327
Omaha, Nebraska 68145
www.AddicusBooks.com

Printed in the United States of America
10 9 8 7 6 5 4 3 2 1

Contents

iii

Part III. My Surgical Approach

To my beautiful children, Andrew, Arianna, Gavin,
and Tallulah. You make every day of my life a dream
and give each day meaning and purpose.
I love you with all my heart.

Acknowledgments

I would like to thank my many friends and colleagues who have assisted me in my development as a surgeon; the American Academy of Facial Plastic and Reconstructive Surgery for its dedication to advancing research and education in plastic surgery; the fellows whom I have trained for their hard work and curiosity, which has helped me continue to evolve as a surgeon; and Dr. Vito Quatela, my fellowship director, for giving me the foundation on which I built my career.

I also thank my dedicated staff, Georgette, Diane, Harriet, Cathy, Joyce, Diana, Nicole, Lana, Cindy, and Peggy, for taking such good care of my patients and me. A special thanks to my patients for urging me to write my second book.

Introduction

My overriding goal as a facial plastic and reconstructive surgeon is to deliver the best natural-looking results with minimal downtime, scarring, and risk for my patients. To that end, I am continuously evaluating my results, then innovating and creating new techniques to improve the outcomes and experience I can offer.

Unlike facial enhancing and rejuvenating procedures of years past, today's methods, I believe, should have the goal not to make everyone look the same, but to unlock the potential that exists in every person's face. This is where science meets art.

In my quest I have found that applying the principles of aesthetic balance from the Renaissance period to plastic surgical treatments has given my patients more-beautiful results while maintaining their identity. By better defining beauty, and applying these concepts to non-invasive, minimally invasive, and more-invasive surgical treatments, the results of plastic surgery leave patients in my practice looking natural, more attractive, more youthful, and more rejuvenated but never manipulated.

My approach combines minimal incision and endoscopic surgery to reposition the deeper facial tissues that droop with age, rather than stretching the surface of the skin, which makes plastic surgery look artificial. For those who want to enhance their beauty by changing the size and shape of their eyes, cheeks, lips, or nose, we combine science with art by employing the principles of the Golden Proportion, which you will read about in chapter 2.

The purpose of this book is to empower you, by providing you with the information you need to make educated decisions about facial cosmetic procedures. It contains in-depth discussions about all of the state-of-the-art lasers, devices, injectable materials, and minimally invasive surgeries available. Specific attention is paid to focusing on what makes a potential patient a good candidate for different treatment, and the benefits and limitations of both nonsurgical and surgical techniques.

Welcome to *The Face of the Future.*

Andrew A. Jacono, MD, FACS
Facial Plastic and Reconstructive Surgeon

PART I.

Characteristics of Beauty

"The greater danger for most of us lies not in setting our
aim too high and falling short, but in setting our aim too low,
and achieving our mark."

—*Michelangelo Buonarroti*

1 The Celebrity Factor

Images of thin, toned, celebrities with "perfect" faces puts enormous pressure on women, starting as early as their preteens. It is no longer good enough to keep up with the Joneses; many younger women feel that they have to keep up with celebrities. But of course that is not realistic. This pressure is not exclusive to women. Men are similarly being held to the celebrity standard; rock-hard six-pack abs and a chiseled jaw and cheekbones are an expectation that is difficult, if not impossible, to meet.

The Ideal Look

The ideal look has changed dramatically over the decades. If you look across cultures and throughout time, beauty standards have certainly evolved, but some aspects of beauty remain constant. For example, the pursuit of symmetry and balance in the face has stood the test of time, even though different ethnicities desire different eyelid, nose, and cheek shapes to maintain their heritage.

Standards of beauty are also very different between the sexes. The beauty ideal for female skin is universally lighter than for males across all cultures. The ideal female face is heart-shaped with a petite jaw, an arched brow, and full lips. Due to a decline in the feminizing hormones estrogen and progesterone as women age, they tend to take on a more masculine appearance. The face becomes square due to cheek volume loss and formation of jowls. Brows flatten, facial hair appears, and lips thin out. The physical traits that can make a man look rugged or handsome tend to make a woman appear more masculine, angry, and tired.

But men are not immune to aging either. Their brows and upper eyelids droop, and lower eyelid bags form, making them look not "rugged" but tired. As the neck loosens, men appear not only older, but also look as if they have gained weight even if they are in good shape.

Focus on Celebrities

Our culture's focus on popular media and celebrity has affected the way we perceive ourselves. A recent study from Harvard University found that "Our society narrowly defines beauty by what we see in entertainment, advertising and fashion runways" so that only 2 percent of women consider themselves beautiful, 5 percent consider themselves pretty, and a mere 9 percent even consider themselves attractive.

This study was based on quantitative data collected from a global survey of 3,200 women from Argentina, Brazil, Canada, France, Italy, Japan, Netherlands, Portugal, the United Kingdom, and the United States. Amazingly, 60 percent of women in this study felt that society expected them to enhance their physical attractiveness. It is no wonder why cosmetic surgery is on the rise! Unfortunately, I do not see our culture changing in the near future, and my goal in this book is to help you to navigate an ever-growing number of options (both nonsurgical and surgical) to enhance your appearance and look great.

While our exposure to beautiful celebrities motivates us to have cosmetic procedures performed on our face, there are other celebrities who make us fearful of making any changes at all. There is no lack of television, movie, and music stars who are examples of "overdone" Botox, fillers injected in the face, and facial plastic surgery. The most common statement I hear is, "If celebrities who have all the money in the world, and the access to the best doctors, look artificial and 'plastic,' what chance do I have at looking good but still like myself after surgery?" The following celebrities are rumored to have had plastic surgery or facial enhancing injections. I split them up into two groups, those who look good and those who look like they "had work done." Some of them have confirmed they had procedures done and some have not; the names are not given in this particular order.

Celebrities who look good as a result of facial cosmetic surgery, are: Madonna, Demi Moore, Susan Sarandon, Ashlee Simpson, Michelle Pfeiffer, Candice Bergen, Kim Kardashian, Julianna Margulies, Jennifer Aniston, Cameron Diaz, and Megan Fox.

In my opinion, the list of celebrities who appear to have had unsuccessful cosmetic surgery and look "done" include: Bruce Jenner, Kenny Rogers, Gary Busey, Joan Rivers, Meg Ryan, Melanie Griffith, Donatella Versace, Heidi Montag, Janice Dickinson, Mickey Rourke, Lindsay Lohan, and Mary Tyler Moore.

It's obvious from this second list that male celebrities walk into these situations as often as women do. Even young celebrities such as Heidi Montag have had procedures done that have left them looking so different from what they did that their look borders on startling. Whether they admit it or not, celebs often don't look "normal" after surgery.

In everyday life many nonfamous men and women also wind up in the same situation. When we look at famous people whose who have had bad results, there are common characteristics of their appearance that make them look manipulated. Using these celebrities as an example we can learn why this happens and how it can be avoided.

Overfilled Lips

One of the most noticeable changes that signal an alteration in celebrities' faces are overfilled lips, especially the upper lip. There are many examples of this, including Meg Ryan, Donatella Versace, Melanie Griffith, and Lisa Rinna for starters. Even young starlets like Lindsay Lohan and at one time Jessica Simpson have fallen victim to these overdone techniques. The filler material can be an injectable product like Restylane, fat transfers, or many others. In an ideal situation, even if one has full beautiful lips, the upper lip should be smaller than the lower lip. In these cases above, that proportion has become reversed. When this happens the entire face becomes unbalanced; it creates an almost apelike appearance with all the focus of the face around the mouth and not on the eyes and cheeks.

The solution to this problem is not to avoid having your lips enhanced (especially if you have thin lips) but to have lip augmentation done correctly, which I discuss in chapter 14. In chapter 4, I discuss how to reverse bad lip injections if your lips don't look balanced.

Overdone Botox

Even a treatment as simple as botulinum toxin injections can leave one looking bizarre. When botulinum toxin is used to reduce wrinkles in the forehead, if the corners of the eyebrows are not treated correctly, they will elevate, leaving you with a "Mr. Spock–like" appearance, similar to the way Jack Nicholson looked in *The Shining*. A picture of the comedian Carrot Top looking like this surfaced in recent years.

When botulinum toxin injections are overdone, it can make the face look downright frozen, like we see in many female newscasters. It has not been confirmed, but I believe that the singer Fergie has had Botox in her forehead that made her eyebrows look heavy and frozen. While she is beautiful, I believe this detracted from her appearance. Botox Cosmetic is a wonder drug, and when used by an experienced injector who understands the facial muscles, it can leave you looking great. I discuss the issues surrounding this treatment in chapter 4.

Overdone Eyelid and Brow Lifts

Some traditional eyelid lift techniques that are routinely performed today change the shape of the eyes and remove all the natural fat around the eyes, making them look sunken. Other examples of altered eyelid appearance are seen in celebrities Bruce Jenner, Gary Busey, and Janice Dickinson.

Additionally, these same celebs appear as if they had an overdone brow lift at the same time that causes a startled appearance. Singer Kenny Rogers's eyes appear startled and sunken at the same time. With these two problems occuring together, these individuals don't look quite like themselves. This does not mean you shouldn't have these procedures done. Techniques that make you look more youthful yet natural are described in chapter 11. Today we can accomplish eyelid and brow rejuvenation without surgery, as will be discussed in chapters 5 and 7.

Overdone Cheekbones

Higher cheekbones are a classic sign of beauty and are seen in the most iconic beautiful women in popular culture, such as Angelina Jolie and Megan Fox. But in their quest to enhance cheeks, many celebrities become so overdone that their faces can look distorted or appear bloated. Certainly they do not look like themselves. Higher cheekbones are accomplished by an experienced physician who injects either a cheek implant or temporary fillers like Radiesse or your own body's fat into these areas.

Melanie Griffith and Joan Rivers are likely to have had overdone fat transfers to their faces, which is why their faces look unusually round and bloated. It has been suggested recently that Lindsay Lohan has had some injectable fillers and fat transfers in her face at the age of twenty-five! Pictures that have circulated of her show her looking "different" and probably ten years older. This demonstrates how when facial filling is overdone it can sometimes actually make a person look older and not younger. I discuss this phenomenon in chapter 2. Many celebrities get facial fillers, but we may not be aware of who does because when done well they look fresh faced and beautiful, not manipulated. Madonna and Cameron Diaz are likely examples of these, even though we have no confirmation they have had anything done. Heidi Montag has admitted to having had large cheek implants. Heidi's case is an example of how overdone implants can even make one's skeletal structure so strong that it masculinizes the face. I will discuss how the cheeks should be properly balanced and proportioned to avoid the "done" look in chapter 13.

Avoiding the "Facelift Look"

The result that no one wants, but many icons acquire, is the stretched look of a more-traditional facelift. Bruce Jenner, Joan Rivers, and Mary Tyler Moore have a classically "facelifted" appearance in which the face appears tight almost to the point of distorting normal facial features such as the mouth. This is generally because the most common technique in face-lifting is to pull the skin up and place some kind of stitching to hold up the underlying muscles of the face. This leaves an excessive amount of tension on the skin, hence it looks pulled or windswept.

Examples of good facelift surgery can be seen in beautiful actresses who seem almost ageless. Although it is not confirmed, it appears that Susan Sarandon, Michelle Pfeiffer, Candice Bergen, and Demi Moore have had exceptionally good surgery. The most state-of-the-art facelift techniques today incorporate less-invasive, small-incision approaches that support the underlying muscles of the face and don't overstretch the surface of the skin. These state-of-the-art techniques are described in chapter 12.

I think that the above examples serve to show how plastic surgery can go wrong, and it is the goal of this book to help you understand how it can go *right*. In upcoming chapters, I discuss all of the procedures available in facial cosmetic surgery. I thank you for taking the journey of reading this book. I know that using it as a resource will allow you to avoid the pitfalls we see in popular culture and help you attain your goals for your appearance. With the help of a great doctor, and there are many out there, you can reclaim your natural beauty that declines with age, and, if you're younger, even enhance the beauty you already have.

References

"The Real Truth About Beauty: A Global Report." Findings of the Global Study on Women, *Beauty and Well-Being*—September 2004, Dr. Nancy Etcoff—Harvard University, Dr. Susie Orbach—London School of Economics, Dr. Jennifer Scott—StrategyOne, Heidi D'Agostino—StrategyOne. Commissioned by Dove, a Unilever Beauty Brand.

2 Where Beauty and Youth Converge: The Golden Proportion

"'Beauty is truth, truth beauty—that is all Ye
know on earth, and all ye need to know."
*—*John Keats*, Ode on a Grecian Urn*

Actress Angelina Jolie is widely considered to be one of the most recognizable and beautiful faces in the world. Beautiful faces such as hers arouse the senses to an emotional level that pleases us. But what are the essential characteristics of a beautiful face? The answer to this question is crucial, especially if a plastic surgeon is going to modify facial features toward a goal of rejuvenating the face and making it appear more attractive. Our goal here is not to make everyone look the same, but to better define the science of beauty so that we can unlock the potential that exists in every person's face.

Interestingly, British researchers asked European white, Asian, and Latino people from a dozen countries to select attractive faces from a diverse collection, and they all chose the same type of faces. Even babies have a sense of what is attractive, as studies have shown that infants three to six months old gaze longer at a nice-looking face than at one that is not attractive.

When we look at a beautiful face, our eyes focus on features that draw highlights and attention, including the eyes, eyebrows, lips, nose, and overall facial shape defined by the cheeks, chin, and forehead. The relative proportion of these features is what can be analyzed and demonstrated to be attractive when proportionate or unattractive when disproportionate.

7

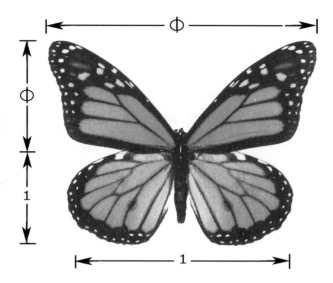

Figure 1. The Golden Ratio is represented in many beautiful things and can be demonstrated in nature in the proportions of a butterfly.

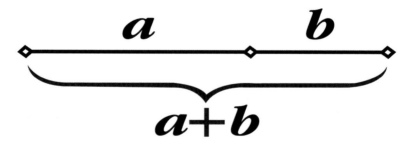

Figure 2. The Golden Proportion, represented by the Greek letter Φ, describes a mathematical relationship between two measurements, which is present in beautiful things (nature, architecture, the human body). If we think of these two measurements represented as a line AB, we can divide it at a point in the line that divides AB in a ratio of 1.618 (A) to 1 (B), or Φ.

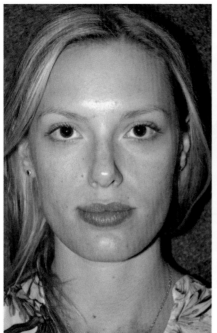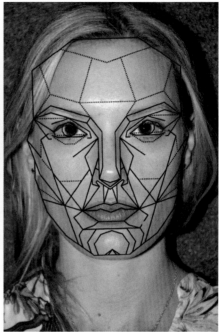

Figure 3. "Marquardt's Golden Mask" represents an ideal face based upon Golden Proportions. When superimposed, notice how this mask conforms to the outline of an attractive woman's face.

Deconstructing the Ideal Face

In looking for what the correct relationship is regarding length and proportion within individual facial features (for example the lips) or the relationship of different features to each other (for example the eyes to the eyebrows), we need to look no further than the Golden Ratio. The Golden Ratio has also been referred to as the Golden Proportion by Renaissance artists, as it has been consistently and repeatedly reported to be present in beautiful things, from architecture to animals to human beings.

The beauty of a butterfly can be demonstrated to have this proportion. Even the structure of a DNA molecule is in this proportion. The Golden Ratio is a mathematical ratio of 1.618:1.0 (this means 1.618 to 1.0) and describes the relationship of one length to another. It is often called Phi (the Greek symbol for Phi is Φ as it was regularly used by the Greek sculptor Phidias. Interestingly, this number is the only one in mathematics that when subtracted by units (1.0) yields its own reciprocal (.618), called phi with a lowercase ϕ, which makes it a uniquely balanced proportion.

9

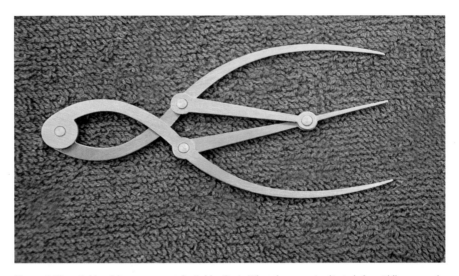

Figure 4. These Golden Calipers represent the Golden Ratio. When the gauge is adjusted, the middle arm marks the Golden Proportion between the two lengths created.

A California-based maxillofacial surgeon, Stephen Marquardt, has derived a perfect face from this Golden Ratio that he refers to as the "Golden Mask," which, when superimposed onto beautiful faces, will routinely match. By superimposing this mask onto a face that lacks aesthetic balance, we can define areas of the face that are deficient or excessive and that can be changed with plastic surgery techniques.

Artists have used the Golden Proportion for more than two thousand years. This has resulted in the development of Golden Calipers that can be used to measure the relationships within and between facial features to create the most beautiful results. I use the calipers when I examine my patients; during injection treatments when trying to create the most beautiful eyebrows, eyes, cheeks, or lips; and during surgery.

Beautiful and natural eyebrow position respects the Golden Proportion (Figure 5). The eyebrow should start at the level of the inner corner of the eye. At this point, the vertical height of the eyebrow should be where the forehead bone starts. The length of the eyebrow should be 1.618 times ϕ, the distance between the inner corners of the left and right eyes. (This is called the *intercanthal distance.*) There should be a gentle upward curve to the brow's lateral tip. The upward curve of the lateral brow tip should be placed .618 times the intercanthal distance above the bone underneath the eyebrow.

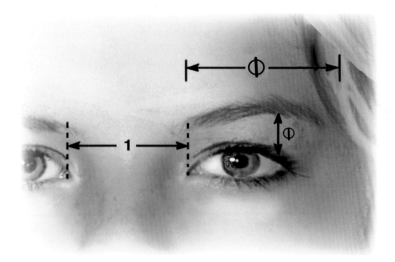

Figure 5. Beautiful eyebrow position is defined by Golden Proportions. $\Phi = 1.618$.

If one does not have eyebrows that have this relationship, they can be changed simply with grooming or makeup. For example, by tweezing the bushiness of eyebrows along their lower edge toward the lateral tip, the Golden Ratio of a beautiful eyebrow tilt is created. Alternatively, an eyebrow pencil can be used to draw a higher brow that respects the Golden Proportion.

Another approach is to perform a brow-lift surgery to tailor its shape. Endoscopic techniques help us control the shape of the eyebrows and not overelevate them, as we will see in chapter 11. Patients are extremely anxious about brow-lift surgery because they see bad results in some people who have had this surgery and now have their eyebrows placed in an overly high position. This gives a deer-in-headlights or startled and surprised look. This look is especially noticeable when the eyebrow position at its beginning is higher or at the same height as its outer tip, not respecting the Golden Tilt of the eyebrow.

The most beautiful eyes have a Golden Ratio between the eyebrows and eyelids. The ratio of the distance from the eyebrow at its highest outer arch to the upper eyelashes is ideally 1.618 times ϕ, the distance from the lower eyelid lashes to the beginning of the cheek (Figure 6). Those with rounder eyes and long lower eyelids have an inverted Golden Ratio and look less attractive. Highlighting the cheeks and lower eyelids with makeup techniques (such as in smoky-eye

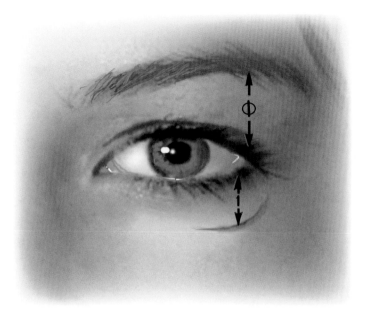

Figure 6. In beautiful, youthful eyelids, the ratio of the length of the upper to the length of the lower eyelids is Φ, or 1.618.

techniques) will shorten the appearance of the lower eyelid and will establish the eyes to a seeming Golden Proportion. This creates a more attractive eye and gives the illusion the eye is more almond shaped.

As we age, our eyelid proportions change. Older brows droop over the eyes, causing the upper eyelid to shorten, throwing off the Golden Ratio. When lower eyelids and cheeks droop, the lower eyelid lengthens, reversing the ideal proportions of the upper and lower eyelids. This droop can be altered temporarily with minimally invasive techniques such as lifting the eyebrows with botulinum toxin (see chapter 4) or shortening the length of the lower eyelid by injecting fillers into the deep eyelid hollows and circles that make the lower eyelids appear longer (see chapter 5). Minimally invasive endoscopic surgery can more permanently lift the brows, and lower eyelid lifts and endoscopic mid-face/cheek lifts can shorten the length of aging lower eyelids (see chapters 11 and 12, respectively).

Beautiful lips also respect Phi. The lower lip should be larger than the upper lip, or, according to this Golden Proportion, the lower lip should be 1.618 times φ larger than the upper lip. The distance from the points of the upper lip, called the peaks of Cupid's bow, to the corner of the mouth should be 1.618 times the distance between the

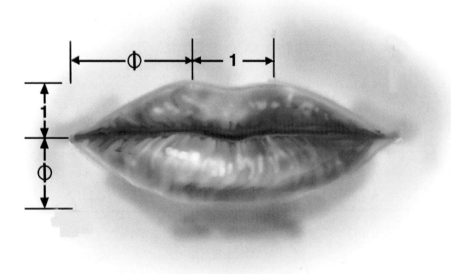

Figure 7. Beautiful lips have Golden Proportions within their structure. $\Phi = 1.618$ and $\phi = .618$.

points of the center of the lip. This is helpful when applying lipstick to create a more naturally beautiful lip that does not look overdrawn. Often, when women apply lipstick, the lips appears artificial if they draw past the lip edges without following these guidelines. When we inject lips with temporary fillers such as Juvederm, we respect the Golden Proportion and do not fill the lips like a shapeless sausage. Surgical lip augmentation procedures that are more permanent, such as lip lifts and V-to-Y lip augmentations are also performed with these measurements in mind, so lips look naturally beautiful and not like a trout pout. When the upper lip is injected larger than the lower lip it has no Phi relationship and is the opposite of the Golden Proportion. I go into more detail in chapter 14.

Beautiful cheeks are defined by their height and volume. We often hear how people desire high cheekbones and appreciate youthful "apple cheeks" that have an oval volume. The ideal location of the cheek can be identified by drawing a triangle around the three major landmarks that surround the cheek. The points of the triangle are from the corner of the mouth to the outer corner of the eye to the center of the ear. The ideal location for a beautiful cheekbone lies along a line drawn from the corner of the eye to the base of this triangle in the Golden

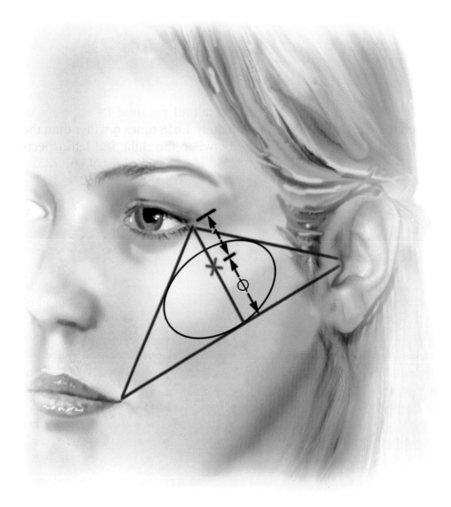

Figure 8. The apex (highest part) of the ideal cheek bone should lie along a line drawn from the base of the triangle (formed from lines drawn from the eye, to the mouth to the ear) to the corner of the eye in the Golden Proportion, $\Phi = 1.618$.

Proportion (Figure 8). Without surgery, this ideal area of the cheek can be accentuated with makeup to make the face more beautiful.

A minimally invasive and temporary way of creating beautiful cheeks is by injecting a filler like Radiesse into this ideal location (see chapter 4). This will make the face more attractive and create the illusion of the entire face being lifted. Creating the Golden Ratio in the cheeks will draw attention to the eyes and cheeks, not to the lower face, making the face more attractive. This result can also be achieved with fat transfers that are more permanent (see chapter 6). Another way to augment the cheeks with implants is discussed in chapter 13.

Youth and Volume—The Heart-Shaped Face

The widest point of the face should be where the cheekbone apex lies, as described above. In a beautiful youthful face the width between the cheekbones is approximately 1.618 times φ wider than the horizontal distance across the face between the right and left aspects of the chin. This creates a "heart-shaped face" with the volume of the face centered around the cheeks. It has a Golden Proportion and is aesthetically more pleasing than older non-"Phied" faces.

As we age, jowls form on either side of the chin, making this horizontal length wider. The cheeks deflate and the distance between them becomes smaller. You can almost think of the young cheek like a helium balloon just after it has been inflated. It is shiny, smooth, round, and full. But as the days go by, the balloon slowly loses helium. Soon the balloon is nothing more than a deflated shell. As deflation of the cheeks occurs, the proportion of the distance between the cheeks and the distance between the lower face along the jawline becomes a ratio of 1 to 1 (equal), and the aging face becomes a square (Figure 9.).

To make the face achieve Phi and restore the natural beauty of youth, a combination of lifting the jowls to reduce the width of the face along the jawline and adding width along the cheekbones is necessary. This can be accomplished in a noninvasive way by tightening the jawline with an Ultherapy treatment (the newest ultrasound jowl-tightening device, discussed in chapter 7, combined with an injectable cheek augmentation as described above. This method usually has temporary results. A more permanent way of re-creating this balance is with a minimally invasive facelift to lift the jowls, narrowing the width of the lower face and lifting the cheeks back up into the center of the face to widen the upper face. These types of procedures will be discussed in chapter 12.

As we continue to age, the cheeks lose more volume and the jowls become heavier, and the face becomes an inverted heart shape, almost like a triangle. Older faces can lose enough volume that lifting the cheeks is not sufficient and volume needs to be added back at the ideal location for cheek augmentation, as noted above. In older faces, it is not enough to simply fill the face because the facial tissues are too loose and cannot support the additional volume. Simply doing a fat transfer for people in their forties can rejuvenate the face without

15

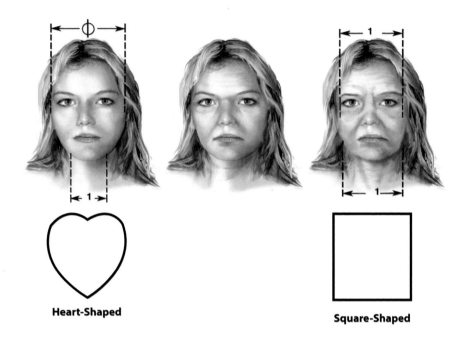

Heart-Shaped

Square-Shaped

Figure 9. Youth is represented by a heart-shaped face with the width along the apex of the cheek bones 1.618, or Φ, the distance between the right and left aspects of the chin. Aging results in deflation of the cheek region and widening of the area around the chin; the formation of jowls creates a more square-shaped face where the ratio between the upper and lower face is 1 to 1.

lifting it, but filling alone for people in their fifties and sixties makes the face take on a more amorphous, overfilled, round appearance. This result looks altered or plastic and is not beautiful. We see this look in many celebrities, as discussed in chapter 1. Although there is no exact age when the face needs to be supported by a lifting procedure, I will discuss what makes you a better candidate for a facelift versus a facial filling procedure in chapter 12.

As you can see, plastic surgery is an art, whether it be a minimally invasive treatment like injections to change the contour of the eyes, eyebrows, cheeks, jawline, or lips, or more invasive surgical procedures. The basic principle of this art is to respect natural proportions that are aesthetically balanced and exist everywhere in nature; this ratio within the face can be described by the Golden Proportion. When art and science do not meet to create such balance, people do not look more beautiful after plastic surgery, but instead look altered and unnatural. What follows in this book is a new approach with the Golden Proportion concept of beauty in mind. We will apply this ratio to all of the most up-to-date, noninvasive, minimally invasive, and more invasive surgical procedures.

References

Jones, D., and K. Hill. 1993. Criteria of facial attractiveness in five populations. *Human Nature.* 4: 271-296.

Lenglois, J.H., L.A. Roggman, R.J. Casey, et al. 1987. Infant preferences for attractive faces: Rudiments of a stereotype? *Developmental Psychology.* 23: 363-369.

Swift, A., and K. Remminton. 2011. BeautiPHIcation™ : a global approach to facial beauty. *Clinical Plastic Surgery.* 38: 347-377.

PART II.

New Minimally Invasive Methods

3 Optimizing Your Skin-Care Program

"Mimicking the fresh luminous skin of youth is not easy, but that hasn't stopped anyone from trying."
—Nancy Etcoff, PhD,
Survival of the Prettiest:
The Science of Beauty

Although I am a facial plastic surgeon, new skin-care products and technologies are available today that provide an alternative to the knife, or at least help us bridge the gap between now and when we are ready to have surgery.

After seeing my patients experiment with countless products and researching every new "cream of the week" to hit the market, I recognize there is no quick fix to aging. You need an ongoing combination of treatments that modify the surface of the skin while addressing the changes brought on by aging in order to alter the canvas of your appearance. The best approach is combination therapies to reverse existing signs of aging and delay future changes for as long as possible.

To understand how to improve our skin, we must first understand the structure of the skin and how it ages. Skin consists of three basic layers, and each of these layers has its own intricate structure. The most superficial layer is the epidermis, the next deeper layer is the dermis, and the deepest layer is the fat layer.

Epidermis

The surface layer of the epidermis is the *stratum corneum* and is composed of dead cells that protect our skin. It is truly like our armor and helps retain our skin's moisture and oil. The stratum corneum is

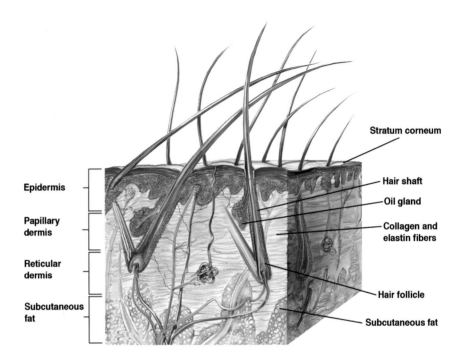

Epidermis

Papillary
dermis

Reticular
dermis

Subcutaneous
fat

Stratum corneum

Hair shaft

Oil gland

Collagen and
elastin fibers

Hair follicle

Subcutaneous fat

Figure 10. The three layers of the skin—epidermis, dermis, and fat layer.

shed continuously and replaced with new cells from the deepest layer of the epidermis called the *basal cell layer*. The other cell type in the epidermis is the *melanocyte* that produces the color and pigmentation of the skin by producing a protein called *melanin*. Caucasians have the same number of melanocytes as African-Americans; however, the melanin concentration in African-Americans is higher. As we age, the epidermis becomes thinner and more disorganized, causing the skin to feel and look rough and dry. Sun exposure accelerates this process.

Dermis

The dermis makes up about 80 percent of the thickness of the skin and is the skin's workhorse and heartbeat. It contains sebaceous glands, hair follicles, sweat glands, blood vessels, and the nerve sensors that allow us to feel touch, temperature, and pain. All these structures are enmeshed in a dense network of *collagen* and *elastin (elastic fibers)*, the primary proteins that support the skin and give it strength and elasticity. The dermis undergoes atrophy with age; elastic fibers degenerate, reducing the resilience and elasticity of the skin, and collagen bulk is lost, causing the skin to become thinner and allowing surface wrinkles to form. Sun exposure causes *dermal elastosis* with further collagen degeneration and disorganization of elastic fibers. Smoking further accelerates the loss of collagen, and the combination of smoking and sun exposure is not additive but synergistic (greater than the sum of the two).

Fat Layer

Under the epidermis and dermis is tissue composed mostly of fibrous tissue and fat. Its function is to insulate the body and further protect the organs, a shock absorber of sorts. This helps keep the skin plump and smooth. Loss of fat as we age results in depressions in skin and causes the skin to sag and fold.

Wrinkle Prevention

Skin ages in two ways: intrinsically and extrinsically. Intrinsic aging relates to all of the things you can't do anything about like genetics, ethnicity, and disease. Extrinsic biological aging, on the other hand, relates to all the things you *can* control, like how much time you spend in the sun, whether you smoke or drink, and how healthy your diet is. This means you are somewhat in control of how your skin will

> Think of these bad lifestyle choices as four major wrinkle generators: sun exposure, smoking, excessive alcohol intake, and poor nutrition.

age. How fast it ages depends largely on how you take care of your skin and the lifestyle choices you make.

There are three ways to prevent extrinsic aging of the skin: 1) avoid skin pollutants/wrinkle generators, 2) protect the skin from daily sun exposure, and 3) supplement and nourish the skin with prescriptive skin care that helps maintain the skin's supple and smooth appearance.

Wrinkle Generators

There are four major wrinkle generators: sun exposure, smoking, excessive alcohol intake, and poor nutrition. Thirty years ago sun exposure was thought to be extremely healthy, so much so that many people applied baby oil/iodine mixtures to the skin to magnify the sun's intensity. It's true that sunlight helps maintain our bodies' levels of vitamin D, an important nutrient, but what we have learned is that all this actinic (sun) damage resulted in an increasing rate of skin cancers decades later, so much so that today the number of newly reported cases is greater than it has ever been in human history. Premature aging of the skin is another side effect of overexposure to the sun. Sun exposure causes a buildup of dead cells in the superficial *epidermal* layer of the skin, giving it the appearance of leather in the most sun-damaged individuals. It also causes *solar elastosis*, a process by which

Three ways to prevent aging of the skin: 1) avoid skin pollutants/ wrinkle generators, 2) protect the skin from daily sun exposure, and 3) supplement and nourish the skin with prescription topical skin-care products that help maintain the skin's supple and smooth appearance.

the collagen and elastin molecules in the deeper dermis of the skin become disorganized and thinned. These changes in the dermis are the direct cause of thinning of the skin and wrinkle formation within the skin.

Too Much Sun

Sun exposure also causes the production of damaging molecules called free radicals in the skin. Our skin cells use oxygen to produce energy, and sunlight causes this oxygen to turn into free radicals that can damage virtually every part of a cell including its DNA. In fact, these scavenging particles are believed to be the major culprit with respect to aging, heart disease, and cancer. Our bodies produces free radicals as part of normal functioning, but sunlight accentuates this production. Antioxidants can be used to prevent the damage free radicals may cause to our skin, both by improving our nutrition and by their application to our skin. I will discuss the ways to use antioxidants to our advantage later in this chapter when we talk about skin care and maintenance.

Smoking

Smoking is another major pollutant of the skin. Smoking has multiple negative effects on the skin. First, the nicotine in cigarettes causes the blood vessels in the skin to constrict and reduce blood supply to the skin which deprives it of nourishment. This chronic skin malnourishment causes all layers of the skin to thin and lose elasticity; as a result, collagen and elastin are lost and wrinkles form. Smoking also causes the release of more free radicals.

Too Much Alcohol

Excessive alcohol consumption causes malnourishment of many essential vitamins and nutrients in our body, including the B vitamin complex and folate, which are essential to skin-cell reproduction and health. Heavy alcohol use also causes free radical production to increase in our bloodstream. This does not mean that a glass of wine with dinner is out of the question. In fact, we have all heard the benefits of moderate consumption of red wine with respect to heart disease. "Moderate" is the key word.

Poor Nutrition

Malnourishment, either as a result of a fast-food diet or from chronic dieting or excessive alcohol intake, decreases the concentration of many antioxidants in our body. Repeat fluctuations in weight as the result of failed diets expands and deflates the skin, resulting in skin that sags more and has more wrinkles. In today's environment it is extremely rare for people to have such severe malnutrition that they deplete their body of essential trace minerals and vitamins, except in the case of alcoholism.

> The newest FDA ruling will make sunscreen manufacturers revise their labeling and many existing products will need to be retested for SPF and broad-spectrum performance. The FDA may also increase the cap of ultraviolet B (UVB) SPF to 50 and up.

Sunblocks

Aside from avoiding wrinkle generators, we need to protect our skin from the sun in everyday life to prevent photoaging. Photoaging is the term for long-term thinning, sagging, and wrinkling that is caused by sunlight. The difference between skin that is photo aged and skin that is just plain aged is the difference between the skin on the face and hands versus the skin on the buttocks. Sunlight contains two kinds of ultraviolet (UV) light: longer UVA rays and shorter UVB rays. UVB rays are the main cause of sunburn and most skin cancers. UVA rays, while not as powerful as UVB, penetrate more deeply in the skin and are the chief culprits behind skin wrinkling and leathering.

The American Academy of Dermatology recommends that a sunscreen or sunblock with an SPF of at least 30 be applied about a half hour before you go outside each day. SPF stands for Sun Protection Factor and measures protection against sunburn-creating UVB (but not

> A study published in 2011 in the Journal of the American Academy of Dermatology found that topical vitamin C appears to provide superior protection from sun damage when used with vitamin E.

UVA). If it normally takes five minutes to get a sunburn on a summer day, a product with an SPF rating of 30 would let you stay outside 30 times longer (150 minutes). Sunblocks that contain zinc oxide and titanium dioxide block UVA rays that cause facial wrinkling; products without these two essential ingredients do not prevent UVA rays as well.

Sun Protection with Topical Antioxidants

Antioxidants may offer protection to the skin and prevent excessive skin aging while nourishing and supplementing its deeper layers. As described above, free radicals cause chronic damage to the cells of the skin, and antioxidants can neutralize these dangerous molecules. Applying antioxidants topically (directly to the skin) is one way of solving the problem of getting additional antioxidants into the skin. However, with topical antioxidants becoming more popular, it is important to know what to look for in a product. Not all antioxidant products contain adequate amounts of antioxidants to have a beneficial effect on your skin. Some of the most effective topical antioxidants follow.

Vitamin C

Vitamin C is vital for producing collagen, which is the substance responsible for giving skin its firmness and elasticity. Vitamin C is also necessary for correcting pigmentation problems and reducing free radicals. It is a water-soluble vitamin that regenerates vitamin E and also provides UVA/UVB protection, decreases pigmentation, reduces redness, and increases collagen production. It also acts as one of the most powerful antioxidants available for skin care and improves the appearance of skin, prevents wrinkles, and is essential in cell proliferation. When you are purchasing vitamin C find out what type and how much vitamin C is in the formula. Be sure that the product you are purchasing is pharmaceutical grade (USP) and tested for highest quality and purity. Be sure the vitamin C is in the form of L-ascorbic acid, which is the only form of vitamin C that the body can effectively use.

Vitamin C is very unstable and unless properly processed and packaged may oxidize before you have the opportunity to put it on your skin. A serum that has turned yellow or brown has oxidized and should not be used. A high-quality vitamin C product will come in a dark bottle to help protect it against oxidation from light. The most common listings are for 10 percent, 15 percent, or 20 percent vitamin C content. For people who have sensitive skin or have never used a vitamin C product before, 10 percent or 15 percent would be a good place to start.

Vitamin E

Vitamin E is a well-known antioxidant with soothing, healing, and moisturizing properties. It is often used to help protect against sun damage and sunburn, to promote healing of burns and cuts, and to improve skin tone. It may also prevent immunosuppression and neutralize free radical damage. Vitamin E's antioxidant properties have been well documented in many studies. In one study when topical vitamin E was applied before exposure to cigarette smoke, the amount of free radicals was cut nearly in half as compared to skin not treated with vitamin E. Vitamin E needs to be in its pure or tocopherol form. Often, cosmetic companies will use a different, less effective form, which does not provide the benefits many consumers associate with vitamin E. A study published in the *Journal of the American Academy of Dermatology* found that topical vitamin C appears to provide superior protection from sun damage when used in conjunction with vitamin E. One reason that the two antioxidants work better when applied together is that vitamin C helps regenerate vitamin E.

Ferulic Acid

Ferulic acid is an organic plant compound found in plant cell walls. It is a potent antioxidant and provides advanced protection from free-radical activity. When combined with vitamins C and E, ferulic acid may reduce oxidative stress. It has anti-inflammatory properties and is effective in neutralizing free radicals. Research has also suggested that ferulic acid may help protect skin from UV damage. Ferulic acid interferes with the process by which UV rays damage cell membranes. In addition, ferulic acid helps to prevent redness and sunburn from UVB rays.

Phloretin

Combined with vitamin C and ferulic acid, *phloretin* creates a potent antioxidant and provides advanced photo protection. It also contributes to greater skin penetration of active ingredients for gradual release and delivery beneath the skins surface.

While there are many over-the-counter preparations, my favorite prescriptive antioxidant skin-care product is SkinCeuticals CE combination antioxidant treatment with 15 percent L-ascorbic acid (the form of vitamin C that's most active in and best absorbed by the skin) and 1 percent vitamin E.

Beauty Diet

I suggest that patients increase their oral intake of antioxidant vitamins and skin-supporting nutrients, in addition to using topical antioxidant therapy, to help protect and nourish the skin. I like to call this the "Beauty Diet." I have listed below the best antioxidants and skin-supporting nutrients to incorporate into your diet. However, to ensure you are getting the appropriate doses daily, it is often best to add them to your daily oral supplement regimen.

Beauty Diet
Six Super-Antioxidants and Nutrients for Aging Skin

- alpha lipoic acid (red meat, brewer's yeast)
- omega-3 fats (fish oils and flaxseed)
- vitamin B5 or pantothenic acid (pomegranates)
- polyphenols (green tea, berries, red wine, chocolate, walnuts, and more)
- vitamin C or L-ascorbic acid (citrus fruits)
- vitamin E (sunflower seeds)

Below I discuss some of the nutrients that I believe are the most effective and easiest to incorporate into a daily regimen.

Alpha Lipoic Acid

Alpha lipoic acid is a fat-soluble and water-soluble antioxidant/anti-inflammatory which allows it to work throughout the body, meaning inside and outside of our body's cells. When taken in supplement form, it may guard against a number of health conditions and also have anti-aging effects on the skin. Dietary sources of alpha lipoic acid include organ meats, red meat, and brewer's yeast. The suggested dosage for antioxidant support is approximately 40 milligrams per day.

Omega-3 Fats

Omega-3 fats are part of a group of essential fatty acids which our bodies are unable to synthesize on their own. Simply put, we are unable to produce omega-3, so it must be acquired from outside sources. In nutrition, important omega-3s include alpha-Linolenic acid (ALA), eicosapentaenoic acid (EPA), and docosahexaenoic acid (DHA). Both DHA and EPA are commonly found in fish oils, while a good source for ALA is flaxseeds. Omega-3s are an excellent anti-inflammatory. Many skin conditions are characterized by inflammation, so anything that helps reduce this is good for the skin. Fish oil has been shown to be an even more effective anti-inflammatory than aspirin and has no serious health side effects. Reducing skin inflammation is an excellent way to improve skin health and reduce specific skin problems. I have observed improvements in skin, hair, and nails when patients incorporate flaxseed and omega-3-rich fish like salmon into their diet. When taking a dietary supplement, 3,000 milligrams per day is suggested.

Vitamin B5

Vitamin B5 or pantothenic acid is found in pomegranates. A study on skin disorders found that topical B5 combats aging and acne by improving skin hydration, maintaining skin elasticity, and increasing skin softness. The study also suggested that B5 has anti-inflammatory properties, making it useful in the treatment of skin scaling, roughness, dryness, and improvement of fine lines and wrinkles; 50 to 100 millligrams daily is suggested.

Polyphenols

Polyphenols are flavonoids found in berries, red wine, olives, chocolate, the skin of grapes, walnuts, and green and white tea, among other substances. They have been studied for their potential positive effects on health including cardiovascular disease, hepatitis, and some cancers. Green tea has been shown to aid in sun damage protection by quenching free radicals and reducing inflammation. Green tea has also been shown to synergistically enhance SPF when used in addition to a sunscreen. Having a cup of green tea each day, whether in the morning or night, is an easy way to incorporate this healthful antioxidant into your nutrition.

The antioxidant properties of vitamins C and E have been extolled above. The recommended daily oral dosing is 1,000 mg per day of vitamin C and 300 IU per day of vitamin E.

Wrinkle Reversal with Topical Skin-Care Products

As we age, our skin develops rough textures, wrinkles, and enlarged pores. When it comes to using topical skin-care products to improve skin appearance, there are two major things that need to be accomplished other than protect and nourish our skin, as discussed above. First, we need to exfoliate and moisturize the surface of our skin, and second, we need to build the deeper collagen layers of the skin that thin with age and even the skin tones and hyperpigmentation.

Exfoliating and Moisturizing

There are two ways to exfoliate the skin: with mechanical exfoliation or chemically with alpha and beta hydroxy acids. Microdermabrasion is a form of mechanical exfoliation that helps slough away the top layer of skin, the stratum corneum, to give it a healthy glow and help increase cell turnover. Usually this device uses crystals that are rubbed over the skin. If you have been to a spa or dermatologist's office for a microdermabrasion treatment, you may have loved that each and every dead skin cell was removed, and you may have benefited from softer skin, less noticeable fine lines, and even a reduction in acne. I would avoid apricot scrubs for routine daily facial exfoliation at home as they have larger, sharp particles that can cause micro-tears to the skin. This can result in premature aging. To avoid expensive visits to the dermatologist, I suggest home microdermabrasion products that use smaller, more delicate particles and a handheld device similar to a dermatologist's microdermabrasion machine but not as aggressive so it can be used daily.

Alpha and beta hydroxy acids (AHAs and BHAs) diminish fine lines and wrinkles. The FDA has approved them as effective to reduce wrinkles, spots, and other signs of aging and sun damage. The more commonly used alpha hydroxy acids include glycolic acid, lactic acid, and ascorbic acid; the beta hydroxy acids include salicylic acid (aspirin-like compound) and benzoic acid.

The first reported use of alpha hydroxy acids was in ancient Egypt. Cleopatra used to take milk baths to add a certain glow to her legendary beautiful skin, and milk contains lactic acid. Alpha and beta hydroxy acids have been demonstrated to decrease the signs of aging

> When it comes to tretinoin therapy, you must suffer the irritation during the initial phase of treatment to attain the ultimate benefits.

by enhancing the shedding of the most superficial layer of the skin, the epidermis. Some claim that these compounds improve the quality of the elastin fibers and the collagen density in the middle layer of the skin, or dermis, thus reversing some of the deeper damage and sagging of the skin.

The effectiveness of an alpha hydroxy acid skin-care product depends mainly on the concentration of alpha hydroxy acids rather than accompanying inactive ingredients with scientific-sounding names.

When prescribed by a physician, the concentration of these compounds ranges from 20 percent to 30 percent. The FDA regulates the concentration of these compounds that can be sold over the counter (OTC). For example, glycolic acid, one of the most popular alpha hydroxy acids, is sold in over-the-counter preparations at concentrations of less than one-fifth the concentration of AHAs that are found in preparations that physicians use, which means the OTC products contain around 5 percent. Products with alpha hydroxy acids concentrated below 8 percent appear to be of no benefit. Most studies of 8–15 percent alpha hydroxy acids report very modest improvements in wrinkles and skin smoothness. A doctor's prescription therefore would result in more significant exfoliation and other positive changes.

Once the skin is exfoliated, it is important to moisturize it. There are many good products available over the counter. You do not need to see a doctor for these. I prefer moisturizers that do not have any other skin-care products included so that they can hydrate the skin without other ingredients preventing penetration. One of the least expensive everyday moisturizers that is available everywhere is Cetaphil DailyAdvance Ultra Hydrating Lotion. The moisturizing formula is fast-acting, long-lasting, and helps moisturize extra-dry skin. It is nongreasy, nonirritating, noncomedogenic (doesn't cause pimples), and fragrance-free. I recommend this product for sensitive, allergenic, and acne-prone skin. It can also be used safely on patients after surgery.

The most expensive moisturizer today is Crème de la Mer, which I have found has wonderful moisturizing properties but costs twenty times what a moisturizer like Cetaphil does. However, I do not think it is twenty times better a moisturizer. Yet I have many patients and even family members who swear by Crème de la Mer. There are many, many other companies that have effective proprietary moisturizers. As long as you moisturize daily, I think any moisturizer is good, so long as it is nongreasy, nonirritating, noncomedogenic, and fragrance-free.

Building the Collagen Layers of the Skin

Vitamin A, peptides, and punicic acid are the three topical agents that have been clinically proven to have the ability to stimulate key constituents of the deeper dermal layers of the skin matrix: collagen, elastin, and glycosaminoglycans (GAGs). Vitamin A was the first vitamin to be used topically for the treatment of damaged skin. The category of vitamin A derivatives includes retinol (vitamin A alcohol) and tretinoin (vitamin A acid). Vitamin A derivatives induce thickening of the epidermis, or outermost surface layer of the skin, increase proliferation of skin cells, and act as a hormone to activate specific genes and proteins in the dermal layers. This hormonal activity increases deposition of new collagen in the dermis, reversing the thinning of this layer that occurs with age.

Topical tretinoin (Retin-A) was the original form of vitamin A that has been studied and proven to accomplish these changes, and it must be prescribed by a doctor. In randomized, prospective, placebo-controlled trials, tretinoin was definitively proven to reduce fine lines and wrinkling, roughness, and laxity. The key to success with Retin-A and other variations is that it should be used consistently. Sunblock must be used daily while on tretinoin, and results take about six months to become noticeable. The biggest problem with Retin-A is that people just do not stick with using it routinely because of its side effects.

Other forms of tretinoin may be less irritating at lower concentrations. Patients who cannot tolerate Retin-A daily are urged to use it every other day or every few days to avoid redness and flaking. Retinol, an alternative to more potent forms of vitamin A derivatives, is universally tolerated in lower concentrations and is available over the counter.

Peptides are essentially chains of amino acids or proteins. Palmitoyl pentapeptide-4 is a skin-rejuvenation peptide that has been included in a variety of commercial skin-care formulas. As mentioned, peptides have been shown to have the ability to stimulate key constituents of the skin matrix: collagen, elastin, and glycosaminoglycans (GAGs). Peptides are reparative when used topically. Some companies claim that the power of peptides in skin-care preparations can mimic

> When it comes to antioxidants, if you can't get the nutrients via your diet, and are on a limited budget, consider a multivitamin that includes some antioxidant-packed nutrients. The effects of antioxidants are very synergistic: certain combinations can enhance the potency of each of the individual components.

the effects of injectable botulinum toxin. This is not true, as no topical cream can penetrate into the facial muscles because they lie deep below the skin. These products work on the lines and wrinkles, but not on the muscles directly. As a consumer, you have to have realistic expectations about the kind of improvements you can achieve with peptides.

Punicic acid is one of the main ingredients in pomegranate seed oil and is effective in cell regeneration and proliferation in the deeper dermis of the skin. Pomegranate seed oil is effective in preventing skin cancer because it is found to reduce lesions and tumors as well. Pomegranate seed oil is mainly known for its nourishing, moisturizing, and protective properties. It is being increasingly used in many lip balms, face creams, lotions, and facial serums. It has been found to be very effective in softening dry, irritated, and aging skin. Pomegranate seed oil activates the growth of keratinocytes (major constituents of the skin's epidermis) and thereby contributes towards the regeneration of the epidermis (outer layer of skin). It is believed to play an important role in the synthesis of collagen, the main fibrous protein of connective tissues. It is also said to retain and improve skin elasticity and reduce the appearance of wrinkles and fine lines.

There are two methods of availing yourself of pomegranate seed oil's skin benefits. You can either opt for cosmetic formulations or use it in its most natural form. Cosmetic creams use an extract of pomegranate seeds and combine it with an array of other chemical ingredients. As a result, most of the properties are lost due to overprocessing. Moreover, these products are often very expensive and do not produce desired results. The best way to get maximum pomegranate seed oil benefits for skin is simply to apply homemade pomegranate seed oil on your skin. Put a handful of pomegranate seeds in a blender to make juice. Strain it and apply it directly on your skin or any affected area. Because no processing or artificial ingredients are involved, the oil's beneficial properties remain intact.

Evening Out Skin Tone

Skin-lightening creams have been around for decades. Lightening the skin or fading away blemishes has been one of the major reasons people use these creams. Historically, the most commonly used ingredient in lightening creams was hydroquinone. It is generally an agent that bleaches the skin. Enzyme reactions that occur in the skin cells are blocked by this product. This results in a slowdown in the creation of melanin which gives skin its color.

Lightening areas of the skin that have darkened is the general use of hydroquinone. Discoloration and darkening of the skin can occur because of melasma, freckles, and age spots. However, the FDA and standards-setting agencies of several countries have cited a skin condition called ochronosis as a concern with hydroquinone use. Although uncommon, particularly with over-the-counter-strength preparations, some people have developed a blue-black skin discoloration after using hydroquinone bleaching creams. Ochronosis also can cause gray-brown spots and tiny yellow-to-brown bumpsas well as skin thickening. Because of these potential dangers, hydroquinone has been banned in Europe. Products containing up to 2 percent hydroquinone are still available over the counter in the United States.

If you are considering using a hydroquinone product on your skin, you should opt for creams with low concentrations of the product, like 1 percent hydroquinone, to reduce your risk.

Because of this potential problem with hydroquinone, newer skin-lightening creams have been developed. Products containing disodium glycerophosphate, L-leucine, phenylethyl resorcinol, and undecylenoyl phenylalanine have been shown in studies to be effective and are alternatives to to hydroquinone to reduce your risk.

References

Fu, J.J., G.G. Hillebrand, P. Raleigh, J. Li, et al. 2010. A randomized, controlled comparative study of the wrinkle-reduction benefits of a cosmetic niacinamide/peptide/retinyl propionate product regimen vs. a prescription 0.02 percent tretinoin product regimen. *British Journal of Dermatology.* Mar; 162(3): 647-654.

Gold, M.H., and J. Biron. 2011. Efficacy of a novel hydroquinone-free skin-brightening cream in patients with melasma. *Journal of Cosmetic Dermatology.* Sep; 10(3): 189-196.

Ho, E.T., N.S. Trookman, B.R. Sperber, et al. 2012. A randomized, double-blind, controlled comparative trial of the anti-aging properties of non-prescription tri-retinol 1.1 percent vs. prescription tretinoin 0.025 percent. *Journal of Drugs in Dermatology.* Jan; 11(1): 64-69.

Leung, Lit-Hung. Pantothenic Acid in the Treatment of Acne Vulgaris: A Medical Hypothesis. *Journal of Orthromolecular Medicine.* 1997; 12.

Morganti, P., C. Bruno, F. Guarneri, et al. 2002. Role of topical and nutritional supplement to modify the oxidative stress. *International Journal of Cosmetic Science.* Dec; 24(6): 331-339.

Murray, J.C., J.A. Burch, R.D. Streilein, et al. 2008. A topical anti-oxidant solution containing vitamins C and E stabilized by ferulic acid provides protection for human skin against damage caused by ultraviolet irradiation. *Journal of the American Academy of Dermatology.* Sep; 59(3): 418-425. Epub 2008 Jul 7.

Oresajo, C., T. Stephens, P.H. Hino, et al. 2008. Protective effects of a topical antioxidant mixture containing vitamin C, ferulic acid, and phloretin against ultraviolet-induced photodamage in human skin. *Journal of Cosmetic Dermatology.* 7(4): 290-297.

Pedrelli, V.F., M.M. Lauriola, P.H. Pigatto. 2011. Clinical evaluation of photoprotective effect by a topical antioxidants combination (tocopherols and tocotrienols). *European Academy of Dermatology/Venereology.* Sep 14. doi: 10.1111/j.1468-3083.2011.04219.

Vranesić-Bender D. 2010. The role of nutraceuticals in anti-aging medicine. *Acta Clinica Croatica.* Dec; 49(4): 537-544.

4 Injection Treatments

Injectable treatments are true medical procedures and should be performed by an experienced physician with detailed knowledge of facial anatomy. A consultation should provide a detailed analysis of your face and a careful review of your goals. For injection treatments, I suggest that patients use a doctor from the core specialties: plastic surgery, facial plastic surgery, oculoplastic surgery, and dermatologic surgery. This will give you the best likelihood of a safe and satisfactory result. Many non-core specialties like pediatricians, OB/GYNs, and even radiologists are trying their hand at these treatments without sufficient training. The risk of complications in these situations goes way up. I discuss how to fix complications from poor injection technique later in this chapter.

There has been a revolution in the number of temporary injectable fillers available in the last decade. For the prior thirty years we had only bovine (cow) collagen injections available. Now there are many different types of molecules to inject, but the main categories of temporary fillers are hyaluronic acid, hydroxyapatite, and poly-L-lactic acid. Because these newer fillers last longer, cow collagen injections are rarely used anymore. In this chapter I discuss the properties of each, where in the face they are best used, and their duration. Later in this chapter I also discuss permanent injectable fillers. In chapter 5, I describe combining different fillers and botulinum toxin treatments to create extreme facial rejuvenation without surgery.

Temporary Wrinkle Fillers

Hyaluronic acid is a sugar-based gel that is injected to diminish folds and wrinkles such as "marionette lines" (the depression below

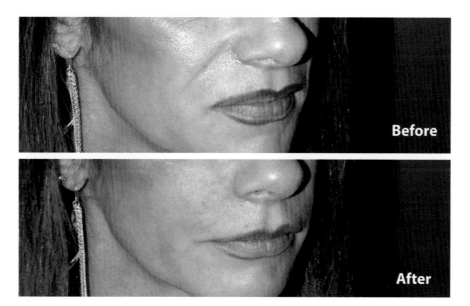

Figure 11. Patient was injected with hyaluronic acid to fill the nasolabial folds, often called "smile lines," between the nose and corners of the mouth.

the corners of the mouth) and "lipstick bleed lines" (the deeper lines that radiate around the lips). This gel also adds volume and rejuvenates the lips, cheeks, under-eye circles, and chins. One of the most common places to have hyaluronic acid injected is in the nasolabial folds, often referred to as the "smile lines" that run between the nose and mouth. Hyaluronic acid is found naturally in our skin, bones, and cartilage. The commercially available products we inject come from a non-animal source and is bioengineered in a lab so there is no need for skin testing like in older collagen preparations. It is a safe compound that is degraded gradually by the body over time.

Juvederm and Restylane are the two most popular dermal fillers in the United States. I have been using both in my practice with great results since they were launched. The duration of effect from hyaluronic acid fillers ranges from six months to one year in most cases. The volume-enhancing effect is created by layering the filler in a series of fine tunnels within the undersurface of the skin. The main difference between these two products is that Juvederm is more stable, and, after injecting hundreds of patients, I have experienced that it tends to last longer. Another main distinction between Restylane and Juvederm is that Juvederm is generally not used around the eyes, as the material tends to absorb water and can make eyes look puffy after treatment in a percentage of patients. For this reason I use only Restylane around the eyes.

Perlane is a sister product to Restylane and is composed of larger hyaluronic gel particles that gives Perlane the additional ability to lift and fill the areas of injection. Because of this property it is frequently used for volume restoration in areas such as cheeks, the pre-jowl sulcus (hollowing on either side of the chin that is accentuated by the formation of jowls), and marionette lines.

The newest hyaluronic acid gel filler to receive FDA clearance is Belotero, which is a finer version of the other products we have available. Belotero may hold certain advantages over the currently available hyaluronic acid fillers due to its ability to treat superficial or fine lines. The other hyaluronic acid fillers noted above can cause a bluish hue if they are injected too superficially. This is called the "Tyndall effect" and represents light reflecting through the skin and bouncing off the clear filler.

Prevelle Silk is another variation of hyaluronic acid, often used for vertical lines around the lip. It tends to have a much shorter duration effect, and more fillers like this are expected to come into the market soon. Some hyaluronic acid fillers, such as Prevelle Lift, are currently awaiting FDA approval in the U.S. market. In Europe there are literally more than one hundred fillers derived from different formulations of hyaluronic acid gels.

One of the main benefits of hyaluronic acid gels is that if the patient wants to reverse the result, such as if too much material is injected, or if the patient has areas of firmness after the treatment, an enzyme called hyaluronidase or Vitrase can be injected to break down the material in a matter of twenty-four to forty-eight hours. In my practice I often dissolve away poorly executed filler injections performed by another doctor. Once the material is removed, I reinject the area of concern more precisely. Experienced injectors have a low number of complications. In chapter 17 I discuss how to choose an experienced physician.

Biostimulators

This category of filling agents works differently from temporary fillers like the hyaluronic acid gels. Biostimulators have the added ability to stimulate new collagen over time. One such material is Radiesse, which is made from the same mineral substance as our bones. Because of its durable nature it lasts longer. Radiesse is made up of microscopic calcium particles (calcium hydroxyapatite) that are suspended in a water-based gel. These microspheres are a very safe material that is used for dental reconstruction, bone growth, and vocal cord injection and is compatible with the body. Radiesse has a collagen-stimulating effect and may produce results that last up to twelve to eighteen months.

Over time, the microspheres degrade naturally into calcium and phosphate ions that are safely metabolized by the body. Radiesse is used in the deepest of the facial folds due to its more viscous nature, but it cannot be injected in the superficial dermis of the skin as it has a white color and shows through. I often use Radiesse to augment the nasolabial folds; lift corners of the mouth; and contour the cheek, chin, and jawline.

Although hyaluronic acids can be used in the same way, I like Radiesse for patients who desire a longer-lasting treatment and do not have time for frequent injection visits. Additionally, I prefer Radiesse in heavier, droopier faces, or when cheeks or other areas of the face need

> Radiesse is used in the deepest of the facial folds due to its more viscous nature, but it cannot be injected in the superficial dermis of the skin as it has a white color and shows through.

more support. The mineral particle of Radiesse is more supportive than hyaluronic acid. One place I use Radiesse more often than any other filler is in the temples. As we get older, starting around age forty, the temple area of the forehead tends to thin and become concave and sunken. Although this area is not as commonly injected as others, when treated at the same time as other portions of the face that droop, it can add significantly to the rejuvenation of the face.

Sculptra Aesthetic is an enduring treatment approved by the FDA for restoration and/or correction of the signs of facial fat loss. It is comprised of poly-L-lactic acid, which is a biodegradable polymer used in suture material. Facial volume loss occurs over time as the soft tissues beneath the skin break down, which can result in sunken cheeks, bony temples, and hollowed under-eye areas. Sculptra Aesthetic is a safe biocompatible material that is injected below the surface of the skin in the area of fat loss. It is not a wrinkle filler, but a bio-activator or volumizer. It works by stimulating the body to produce new collagen at the sites of injection, thereby replacing lost volume

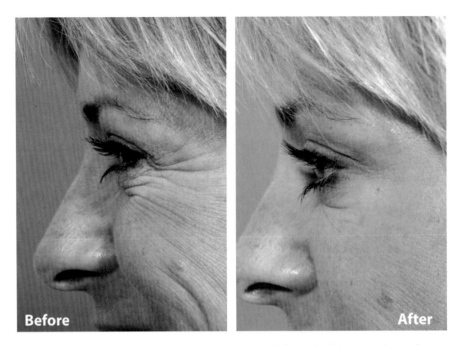

Figure 12. This patient injected with botulinum toxin to soften the "crow's feet" that occur when smiling.

and contours to restore a fuller, more youthful appearance. It is not useful for more-superficial lines and folds. Typically, a series of two or three treatments of Sculptra Aesthetic is needed to achieve optimal outcome that can last for up to three years in some cases.

While the longevity of this treatment is the best of all the injectable treatments, there are drawbacks. Sculptra Aesthetic requires three separate injection sessions instead of one (as with hyaluronic acids or Radiesse), so there is a greater financial investment up front.

Wrinkle Relaxers: What Botulinum Toxins Do

Wrinkles are in many cases the direct result of contraction of delicate facial muscles underneath the skin surface. This causes the overlying skin that is attached to the facial muscles to wrinkle and fold. Examples of this are the wrinkles around the eyes called the "crow's feet" that result from our smiling, vertical lines between the eyebrows called "11s" or "frown lines" that occur when we concentrate or are angry, and the horizontal forehead wrinkles that happen as a part of normal daily facial animation. You do not have to be a facial plastic surgeon to realize that the way we treat these lines of motion is to stop the muscles from contracting. This results in a flattening of the overlying skin.

Botulinum toxin is a medication injected into the muscles that works by blocking the nerve impulses to the wrinkle-producing muscles so they do not contract. Botox Cosmetic (onabotulinumtoxinA) is the most widely used botulinum toxin treatment for this problem and the first to gain FDA approval. As a result, the overlying skin will be smooth and unwrinkled. The untreated muscles will allow for normal facial expression to remain unaffected. I administer very precise injections into the areas selected for treatment. The treatment is simple and with minimal discomfort—people often get treated during their lunchtime—and you can immediately resume normal activity.

Botulinum toxin is the most common injectable treatment that I administer in my practice. People always ask whether they will feel frozen after the treatment, but the medication does not change the sen-

> Don't shop for the cheapest Botox. When physicians offer discounts on these treatments, it is often because the Botox has been heavily diluted. That means it will last for a shorter period of time. If the treatment sounds cheap, you may not be getting what you think you are.

sation of the skin, it just stops the muscles from moving. Patients also are concerned that botulinum toxin injections are somehow addictive, but this is not the case; you get about as addicted to botulinum toxin as you do to your hair color. Just as when you start to see your root color come back you get a touch-up; similarly, when your wrinkles come back you get a "touch-up." It takes forty-eight to seventy-two hours before the effect starts to take place, and full penetration of the botulinum toxin can take up to one week. Sometimes a touch-up may be necessary to even the result at one week posttreatment.

You will still be able to laugh, smile, or frown, but without the wrinkles. The duration of effect is between four and six months, and long-term maintenance can be achieved by repeated treatments.

Botulinum toxin has been used in medicine for over two decades to treat spastic muscular disorders and is extremely safe. Complications are quite rare, unless the treatment is improperly administered or too much is used in the wrong place. This problem will be discussed in the section below, "When Good Temporary Fillers and Botox Go Wrong and How to Fix Them."

Two other forms of botulinum toxin are Dysport and Xeomin. Dysport (abobotulinumtoxinA) is so similar to Botox Cosmetic that it is referred to as Botox Cosmetic's twin or first cousin. This new wrinkle relaxer is approved in the United States to treat forehead wrinkles and frown lines. Exactly how the two wrinkle relaxers differ is not fully understood. Studies show that Dysport acts quicker. Botox Cosmetic takes three to five days to work, while Dysport works within one to two days. In some cases, wrinkles begin to fade as soon as twenty-four hours after receiving Dysport treatments. This rapid response could be the deciding factor for women or men looking to improve their appearance before a big social event or meeting. In my experience, the original Botox Cosmetic and Dysport have a similar length of duration, and they can both deliver great results by an experienced injector.

The latest contender in a growing list of botulinum toxin injectables is Xeomin (incobotulinumtoxinA). The Food and Drug Administration (FDA) approved Xeomin in July 2011 for the treatment of severe frown lines or "11s" between the eyes. Xeomin is also "naked," meaning that there are no additives, just botulinum toxin type A. This may mean that there is less risk of developing antibodies against Xeomin than other available neurotoxins. This is important because antibodies help the body digest the botulinum toxin so its effects on the face fade away. The full effects of Xeomin occur within one week, and the results last from three to six months, making it comparable to Botox in terms of both onset and duration of action.

Other Uses for Botox

Botulinum toxins can also be used to lift the eyebrows, reduce marionette lines, and relax the cords in the neck, among other uses (see Table 1). These are considered "off-label" uses, which means they are not FDA-approved for that use. Botulinum toxins are FDA-approved to be used only in the frown lines between the eyebrows. However, botulinum toxins are used in an off-label way routinely in the United States. Although FDA approval is specific as to a drug's intended use, physicians are able to decide how to best prescribe, use, and/or administer a drug or device.

The way to understand how botulinum toxin lifts portions of the face is to understand that there is a constant tug-of-war going on in any section of the face. There are muscles that lift a portion of the face (for example the eyebrow) and opposing muscles that pull it down. If we inject Botox in the muscle that pulls things down, the muscle that lifts wins, and the result is that that portion of the face is elevated.

Table 1. "Off-Label" Facial Treatments with Botulinum Toxin.

Facial Area Treated with Botox	How it Works
Neck Bands and Cords	Thick bands on the front of the neck called platysmal bands can be softened with botulinum toxin in a subtle way. This technique works best on thin necks where the muscle bands are most obvious when chewing and grimacing.
Brow Lift	The muscles that pull down the eyebrows include the corrugator supercilli muscle between the eyebrows and the orbicularis muscle at the outer tail of the brow. Injecting these sets of muscles with different quantities of toxin not only allows the brows to lift, but a good injector can shape and tilt the brows.
Drooping Corner of Mouth, Frowning	Turning up the corners of the mouth is accomplished by injecting the muscle called the depressor anguli oris, which pulls the corner of the mouth down. Preventing it from contracting releases the frown and allows it to turn up.
Nonsurgical Nasal Tip Lift	A droopy tip of the nose can be cause by an overactive muscle called the depressor septi muscle that pulls down the nasal tip. Botulinum toxin can be injected in between the nostril on the undersurface of the nose to release the tip and create a more upturned nose.
Chin Dimpling	Too many chin dimples can be caused by an overactive chin muscle called the mentalis. This condition is called a *peau d'orange* chin because it looks like the surface of an orange. The chin will look smoother after a few units of botulinum toxin is injected.
Gummy Smile	A gummy smile is created by hyperactive muscles called the lip elevators which make the teeth too exposed. The muscles injected are the levator labii superioris and levator labii superioris alaeque nasi, which prevents the lip from elevating too much so much that it shows the gums during a smile.

Facial Area Treated with Botox	How it Works
Pore Size	Botulinum toxin has been found to be helpful for acne sufferers. Injections made just under the skin affect the sebaceous or oil glands, which are the culprits behind oil production. Pore size can appear reduced and acne breakouts are diminished.

When Good Temporary Fillers and Botox Go Wrong, and How to Fix Them

Some of the most common problems I see with injectable filler treatments are overinjected areas and firmness or lumps that occur after the injection. This can occur anywhere fillers are injected. Cheeks, lips, and eyelids can be overfilled, causing the face to look plastic and sometimes even distorted. Bumpiness and lumpiness can occur if too much of the product is injected in one spot or if the filler is injected too superficially in the skin. Depending upon the type of temporary filler used, these problems may or may not be reversible, so certain fillers should not be injected in certain areas.

When the hyaluronic acid fillers (i.e. Restylane, Juvederm, Perlane, Belotero, Prevelle Silk) are overinjected, the material can be dissolved away with hyaluronidase or Vitrase, an enzyme that will make the implant disappear in twenty-four to forty-eight hours. Sometimes more than one treatment needs to be performed to remove all the material injected, and these treatments should be separated by a week or two.

Radiesse and Sculptra Aesthetic are more likely to create nodules. Radiesse contains a gel, to aid in injecting it, which is reabsorbed after three weeks. If nodules develop, patients should massage the area to make the gel dissipate quicker than three weeks. If this does not work, an experienced doctor can try to break it up by using an 18-gauge needle which will allow the body to reabsorb some of the Radiesse. Since Sculptra Aesthetic creates collagen-like tissue from your body reacting to the poly-L-lactic acid injected, reducing your body's reaction to the material can reduce any nodularity. This can be accomplished by injecting a steroid called Kenalog, often used by dermatologists to control pimples and cysts, in dilute amounts. Another method of camouflaging uneven or irregular areas where Radiesse and Sculptra Aesthetic have been used is to inject a hyaluronic acid like Restylane or Juvederm over the area so it looks smoother as the filler dissolves on its own over time.

The lips are one of the areas that are most overdone with fillers. The results are often referred to as "duck lips," "sausage rolls," and "trout pouts." It is important to never inject Radiesse or Sculptra Aesthetic for lip augmentation because they tend to form hard, painful nodules that can take up to a year to go away. The best filler option for lips is hyaluronic acid.

The reason lips can look odd after treatment is that either the lips were overfilled, or the aesthetically pleasing proportion of the lip that is governed by the Golden Ratio was not respected. The Golden Ratio was discussed in chapter 2. According to this proportion, the lower lip

The two most techically difficult areas of the face to treat well with fillers are the lips and the tear troughs under the eyes.

should be 1.618 times larger than the upper lip. The distance from the points of the upper lip, called the peak of Cupid's bow, to the corner of the mouth should be again 1.618 times the distance between the points of the center of the lip. Overfilled lips have improper proportions. To correct this, the material can be dissolved away with hyaluronidase or Vitrase, an enzyme that will make the implant disappear in twenty-four to forty-eight hours.

Another area that can have problems when injected by less-experienced doctors is the eyelids. Sculptra Aesthetic and Radiesse should not be injected around the eyes because these materials cause nodules in this part of the face. The dark circles or sunken area of the lower eyelids should be injected only with hyaluronic acids. The lower eyelids are composed of very thin skin and injecting these fillers too superficially can often result in visible lumps, nodules, and irregularities. As mentioned earlier, one such problem is called the "Tyndall effect" and represents light reflecting through the skin and bouncing off the clear filler. This can be avoided by using either Restylane or Belotero in this area, both of which have less tendency to the "Tyndall effect" , and by injecting the material deeper. Juvederm has more of a tendency to the "Tyndall effect" and should be avoided, and Perlane is harder, so it can create more lumps in the thin eyelid skin.

If redness, prolonged swelling, tenderness, or hardness persist after injections, this can be a sign of an infection called a biofilm. Biofilms can form even when the appropriate injection material is used and surgery is performed by an expert physician injector. A biofilm is basically made up of bacteria that are stuck to each other and/or to the injected filler material. Biofilms can also form in breast implants and cheek implants. The reason biofilms can be problematic is that they are resistant to antibiotics and tend to persist, thus spreading infection. The best way to deal with biofilms is to prevent them in the first place.

Therefore, a high standard of care should be used to prevent infection, such as cleansing the skin with antiseptics before the injection. If a biofilm does occur, a combination of the oral antibiotics Biaxin and Ciprofloxacin along with Vitrase injections is in order.

Many patients are fearful of looking frozen or odd after botulinum toxin injections. There is good reason for this fear. Many people we see in everyday life look "Botoxed." One of the most common places that botulinum toxin injections have problems is in the forehead. When too much Botox is placed in the horizontal lines of the forehead, it is

> Notify your doctor right away if you feel increasing tenderness that develops after a filler treatment because it might be a biofilm infection, and early treatment can be helpful.

impossible to lift the eyebrows. This can make you look frozen, like many newscasters who appear expressionless. It also can make your eyebrows fall over your eyelids, making them look droopy. Once this happens there is no way to fix the problem; it usually takes four to six weeks for the botulinum toxin injections to wear off to the point where your eyes are not as droopy, but the forehead lines are still corrected.

Another problem that can occur in the forehead is "Mr. Spock eyes." This can occur when only the center of the forehead is treated with injections and the eyebrows are lowered. Since the outer corner of the eyebrows can still move, they point up. This is the look Jack Nicholson had in the movie *The Shining*. As noted in the chapter 1, the comedian Carrot Top has been photographed with this appearance (even though it has not been confirmed that he used botulinum toxin). This problem can be corrected by injecting a small amount of botulinum toxin in the forehead above the area where the eyebrows lift.

If a botulinum toxin migrates into the upper eyelid from injections placed around the eyes or eyebrows, a condition called blepharoptosis can develop. Blepharoptosis is when the muscle that opens the eye, the levator muscle, gets weakened. This makes one eye look droopy like you have had a stroke. This problem happens in about only 0.1

percent of patients in an experienced injector's hands. I have seen it in patients who have been injected by other doctors, for example a radiologist, who were not well trained in this treatment. The only remedy for this is to use eye drops called iodipine that will make the eye open. It can help you function socially during this difficult time. Unfortunately, the medicine works for only an hour or two at a time and, if overused, the drops stop working. The problem usually improves after six weeks as the effects of the botulinum toxin begin to wear off.

The Hidden Dangers of Permanent Fillers

Permanent facial fillers seem like a great idea because they prevent the need for repeat visits for temporary filler injections which are time-consuming and expensive. The only FDA-approved permanent filler for use in the face is Artefill, but the most commonly injected permanent facial filler in America is liquid silicone, which is not FDA-approved. There are many other permanent fillers that are used around the world and I will discuss some of these below, but they are not commonly used in the United States because many have high rates of complications, and they are not FDA-approved.

For more than fifty years, liquid injectable silicone has been used for soft tissue augmentation, drawing polarized reactions from both the public and from physicians. While many doctors consider silicone too risky for facial cosmetic injections, it can be used safely if injected by an experienced professional who uses an appropriate medical injecting-grade silicone. This is called an "off-label" use as liquid silicone is approved only to be injected into the eyeball to treat a detached retina, but not the face. Because liquid silicone is used as a lubricant for hypodermic needles, it is technically being introduced in tiny amounts every time anyone receives an injection of any kind. While I do not perform liquid silicone injections, I have seen many patients who have had these injections done by my colleagues and have good results.

As I have mentioned, Artefill, a mixture of synthetic beads of polymethyl methacrylate, or PMMA, mixed with bovine or cow collagen, is the only FDA-approved permanent facial filler. After the collagen reabsorbs, the synthetic PMMA microspheres in ArteFill are nonresorbable, stimulating the body to generate its own natural collagen to encapsulate each individual microsphere. After the collagen component dissipates, these beads permanently fill the wrinkles injected. An allergy test is usually done about a month before treatment because some people can be allergic to the cow collagen in Artefill.

Bio Alcamid was previously available in Canada and Europe and presented some severe complications for patients. It is an injectable water-based polyalkylimide gel containing a small percentage of polyalkylimide. It was used to treat soft-tissue defects and build up volume in the face, but it was also used in some cases for the cheeks, chin, and lip augmentation. It is nonbiodegradable, doesn't reabsorb, and forms a collagen capsule around it. I have never injected it, but I have done surgery on many patients who have had problems with the material. The most common complication I have seen with Bio Alcamid is that it seems to build up in one area typically years after injection. Another complication is hardening of the capsule of collagen

> All permanent facial fillers have three major risks:
> formation of permanent granulomas/nodules, migration, and the in-ability to be removed without surgery if you are having problems or do not like the way they look.

surrounding the implant. These changes cause a visible and disturbing disfigurement for patients that can be corrected only with surgery.

All permanent facial filler injections have three major risks that cannot be easily reversed: overinjection, granulomas, and migration. The most notable complication is overinjection of large volumes of permanent fillers which can result in distorted features like rounded faces, swollen cheeks, or large lips. This can be avoided when performed by highly experienced physicians. What cannot be controlled by any physician, no matter how expert he or she is, is that a small percentage (1 to 3 percent) of patients will develop a chronic reaction against the material and form nodules called granulomas, or that the material will migrate. When granulomas occur the doctor may try to inject a dilute steroid called Kenalog to try to prevent the rejection, but this often fails. Migration is the third problem that can occur, meaning the injected permanent filler can move away from the intended site. This does not usually happen initially, but after many years (ten years or more) the facial tissues loosen and lose thickness. The filler can show through this thinner skin, even though it never did in years past.

If these problems occur, the only way to correct them is to remove the material. This requires an incision on the face that can leave a scar. I perform a lot of revision surgery on patients who have had complications from permanent filler injections, so I am reluctant to inject these materials.

References

Bass, L.S., S. Smith, M. Busso, et al. 2010. Calcium hydroxylapatite (Radiesse) for treatment of nasolabial folds: Long-term safety and efficacy results. *Aesthetic Surgery Journal.* Mar; 30(2): 235-238.

Dayan, S.H., J.P. Arkins, R. Brindise. 2011. Soft tissue fillers and biofilms. *Facial Plastic Surgery.* Feb; 27(1): 23-8.5.

Nettar, K.D., K.C. Yu, S. Bapna, J. Boscardin, C.S. Maas. 2011. An internally controlled, double-blind comparison of the efficacy of ona-botulinumtoxinA and abobotulinumtoxinA. *Archives of Facial Plastic Surgery.* Nov-Dec; 13(6): 380-386. Epub 2011 Jun 20.

Prager, W., V. Steinkraus. 2010. A prospective, rater-blind, randomized comparison of the effectiveness and tolerability of Belotero® Basic versus Restylane® for correction of nasolabial folds. *European Journal of Dermatology.* Nov-Dec; 20(6): 748-752. Epub 2010 Oct 26.

Vartanian, A.J., A.S. Frankel, M.G. Rubin. 2005. Injected hyaluronidase reduces Restylane-mediated cutaneous augmentation. *Archives of Facial Plastic Surgery.* 7(4): 231-237.

5 The Art of Injectable Rejuvenation

As a facial plastic surgeon who had few options other than a surgical procedure for my patients ten years ago, I am excited about the number of new injectable treatments that have become available and are useful in my daily practice. They have given my patients the freedom to rejuvenate their appearance while continuing to work and engage in their personal lives, as there is essentially no downtime. Interestingly, I find that many patients will have these treatments performed around the time of important events to look refreshed and camera-ready, for example when their children are getting married.

While injectable treatments never give results that are as beautiful or dramatic as surgery, they help us bridge the gap between now and when we are ready to have surgery. In chapter 7 we will look at other options to help turn back the clock without surgery. Here I will discuss the use of a combination of injectable treatments covered in the chapter 4 to create results that are similar to more invasive surgeries like a facelift, eyelid lift, or rhinoplasty; that is why they are commonly referred to as liquid facelifts, nonsurgical eyelid lifts, and nonsurgical nose jobs. The term "liquid facelift" has been popularized in the media over the last five years. Interestingly, it is somewhat of a misnomer because the majority of injected materials are not liquid at all. Hyaluronic acids and biostimulators are semisolid so they can reshape the face, eyes, and nose by supporting different facial tissues. This is something a liquid cannot do.

The Liquid Facelift

To understand how the liquid facelift works, we must first understand the nature of facial aging. As discussed in chapter 2, you can almost think of the young cheek like a helium balloon just after it has been inflated. As it is deflated, the balloon is nothing more than a deflated shell. As this deflation of the cheeks occurs, the face goes from being a heart shape to being a square. This means the distance between the cheeks and the distance between the lower face along the jawline become equal. Refilling the cheeks will lift them like a reinflated balloon and reestablish the heart shape.

The location at which we fill the cheeks is critical. The correct location to reinflate cheeks so they look beautiful is at the upper third of the face at a point that represents the intersection of the Golden Ratio of Beauty of 1.618 to 1 (see figure 8 in chapter 2). The injections are placed deep over the cheekbones, supporting the face more than

> Refilling the cheeks will lift them like a reinflated balloon and reestablish the heart-shaped face of youth.

if just injected into the skin. When injections are placed in the middle of the cheek on either side of the nose, people look almost apelike. They may not look droopy but they don't look beautiful. My favorite injections to use for this area are Perlane, Radiesse, and Sculptra Aesthetic as they tend to be denser and more supportive of the face than other fillers.

As part of the liquid facelift, the jowl and jawline can be lifted with a combination of supportive filler injections and botulinum toxin injections. The jawline can be supported by using deep fillers over the jawbone underneath the jowling area. Again, I prefer Perlane, Radiesse, and Sculptra Aesthetic for these treatments. The marionette lines that begin at the corner of the mouth and end at the chin in front of the jowl are also filled just under the skin. Here it is more common to use Juvederm or Restylane which are softer and cause less lumpiness. To help lift the neck and marionette lines, botulinum toxin treatments are added. Thick bands on the front of the neck called platysmal bands can be softened with botulinum toxin in a subtle way. Marionette lines are further improved by injecting botulinum toxin into the muscle called the depressor anguli oris. This muscle pulls the corner of the mouth down, so when it is released with botulinum toxin the corner of the mouth lifts.

The end result is a rejuvenated appearance that can make you look five to ten years younger without surgery or significant downtime.

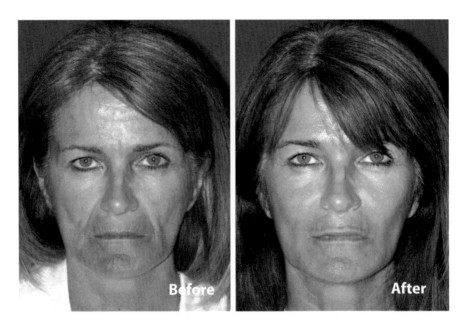

Figure 13. Patient had a "liquid facelift" to non-surgically lift the face. Radiesse and hyaluronic acid fillers were used to lift the cheeks, add volume to the face, and reduce the folds around the lower face and mouth.

Liquid facelifts yield the best results in patients in their forties to sixties. There are two downsides to this approach, however. The first is that it is temporary fix, requiring one or two injection sessions a year. This can get very time-consuming and expensive. These treatment sessions require multiple vials of filler and botulinum toxin and, as a patient, you pay a fee for each vial that is used. In fact, it is not uncommon to spend the same amount of money in three years as it would cost for surgery, and surgical procedures that lift the face generally last ten years. Another disadvantage is that as we get older and and our face gets droopier, we need more and more vials of injectable material, and the injections provide less improvement. It is usually at this point that many patients decide to opt for surgery. There is no perfect age or perfect time for surgery; I have patients who have surgery in their forties and some in their seventies. It simply depends on how much improvement you are looking for and the cost and time involved.

Nonsurgical Eyelid Lift

To understand how an eyelid lift can be accomplished without going under the knife, we must first consider the aspects of youthful eyes and how they change with age. Ideally, the ratio of the distance from the eyebrow at its highest outer arch to the upper eyelashes is 1.618 times the distance from the lower eyelid lashes to the beginning of the cheek. This is the Golden Proportion or Golden Ratio. As we age our eyelid proportions change. Older brows droop over the eyes, causing the upper eyelid to shorten, throwing off the Golden Proportion of youth. When lower eyelids hollow and cheeks droop, dark circles under the eyes are created.

The "nonsurgical eyelid lift" uses injectable treatments to reestablish youthful proportions and rejuvenate tired eyes. A combination of the reshaping properties of botulinum toxin and temporary fillers is often used. Botulinum toxin is injected into the muscles that pull down the eyebrows, including the corrugator supercilli muscle between the eyebrows and the orbicularis oculi muscle at the outer tail of the brow. Injecting these muscle sets with different quantities allows the brows to lift, opening the upper eyelids and reestablishing the Golden Proportion of the upper eyelid. A good injector can shape and tilt the outer brows. The dark circles or sunken areas of the elongated lower eyelids

> As we age, our eyelid proportions change. Older brows droop over the eyes, and lower eyelids hollow and cheeks droop, creating dark circles under the eyes.

should be injected and filled only with hyaluronic acids. This shortens the distance from the lower eyelashes to the cheek and reestablishes the Golden Proportion. Since the lower eyelids are composed of very thin skin and injecting these fillers too superficially can often result in visible lumps, nodules, and irregularities, it is wise to have this procedure done by an experienced injector.

Many patients will start with nonsurgical eyelid lifts in their thirties when these changes start to occur and continue with them into their late forties. Around their fifties the tissues of the eyes become loose and droopy enough that the injections have less of an effect, and this is when patients will usually have surgical eyelid lifts performed. This procedure is less expensive than a liquid facelift because the area around the eye is smaller and requires fewer vials of material.

Nonsurgical Nose Jobs

"Nonsurgical nose jobs" (nonsurgical rhinoplasties) are performed using injectable fillers and botulinum toxin to restore a more symmetric

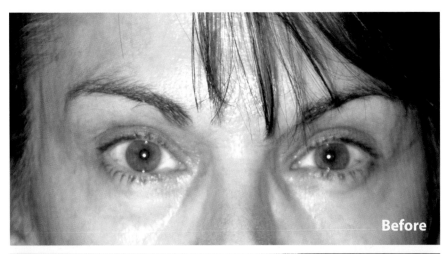

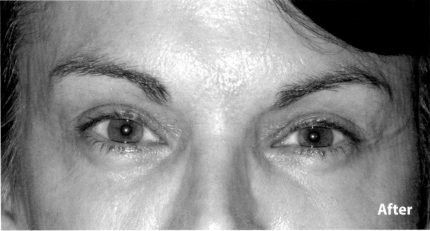

Figure 14. Patient who had a "nonsurgical eyelid lift." Botulinum toxin was used to lift the brows and open the eyes. Hyaluronic acid injections were used to fill the dark circles under the eyes and to reduce the appearance of lower eyelid bags.

look to your nose. Controlled and precise injections can make the nose look more proportional and smaller in the facial frame. The results are instantaneous and there is essentially no recovery time, unlike surgery. The most common filler used is Radiesse, which is made up of calcium hydroxyapatite crystals that are very similar to the mineral found in the bones of the nose. It is also ideal because it lasts approximately one year, which is twice as long as most other fillers (hyaluronic acids) that we have available. Although nonsurgical nose jobs are a welcome alternative to surgery, there are limitations to what this approach can accomplish. I will discuss this below. The surgical approach will be discussed in chapter 15.

The are many ways we can reshape the nose with fillers. The most common way we use injectable fillers is to diminish the appearance of bumps on the nose. By injecting the bridge above the bump, it makes the nose appear straighter. This cannot, however, make a bridge smaller, or create the gentle, feminine curve in the bridge that many women desire. I stress this difference to patients as I have seen many people treated by other physicians who have oversold this procedure as "removing the bump." While these patients described their nose as appearing straighter, they said it did not make it smaller which is what they expected; most patients who have a bump on the bridge don't come in requesting a straighter bridge but want the bump gone. I think injectables can be a wonderful treatment as long as the patient understands what the procedure will accomplish and has realistic expectations.

In other patients who have a flat nasal bridge, injecting fillers will create or augment the bridge. This is a very common request in the Asian and African-American population who often have flatter noses. Unlike the situation with nasal humps described above, this treatment can give results similar to rhinoplasty surgery because the surgery uses either your own cartilage or a permanent implant to build the bridge instead of a temporary injection. The difference between surgery and the nonsurgical approach is simply that surgery gives a permanent result that does not require repeat treatments.

The nose can be further reshaped by filling in dents, hollows, or indentations. In patients who have had a prior rhinoplasty surgery and still have irregularities, using a filler can be a welcome alternative to undergoing a more complex revision rhinoplasty surgery. This is especially true if the imperfections after surgery are minor (like small depressions in areas around the tip and bridge) and only small refinements are necessary.

Many patients want the droopiness of their nasal tip to be lifted with injections. A droopy tip of the nose can be caused by an overactive muscle, the depressor septi muscle, that pulls down the nasal tip, especially when an individual smiles. Botulinum toxin can be injected in between the nostrils on the undersurface of the nose to release this muscle and create a more upturned nose. This result will usually last three to five months. Fillers can be added where the nose meets the lip to support the tip at its base. Using both of these techniques together gives the best results, but the reality is that it lifts the tip by 2 to 3 millimeters in the best cases, which is not very much. Because of this, the nonsurgical approach is best reserved for patients who require only a small amount of lifting of the tip. Those with heavy or droopier tips will not usually not see a significant difference to make it worth the expense, so surgery is a better option here.

References

Humphrey, C.D., J.P.Arkins, S.H. Dayan. 2009. Soft tissue fillers in the nose. *Aesthetic Surgery Journal.* Nov-Dec; 29(6): 477-484.

Morley, A.M., and R. Malhotra. 2011. Use of hyaluronic acid filler for tear-trough rejuvenation as an alternative to lower eyelid surgery. *Ophthalmologic Plastic and Reconstructive Surgery.* Mar-Apr; 27(2): 69-73.

Schierle, C.F., and L.A. Casas. 2011. Nonsurgical rejuvenation of the aging face with injectable poly-L-lactic acid for restoration of soft tissue volume. *Aesthetic Surgery Journal.* Jan; 31(1): 95-109.

6 The Stem Cell Facelift, Volume Restoration with Fat Transfer, and the Vampire Facelift

As a culture we value the firm, round, nubile skin of youth. But as we age, we lose the fat that makes young skin look full. We also lose collagen and elastin that gives skin its firm and elastic quality. The more fat, collagen, and elastin we lose, the looser the skin gets and the more it starts to sag.

The Stem Cell Facelift

A "stem cell facelift" is a misnomer since it does not actually lift the face like a traditional facelift. It is a procedure that utilizes fat that is suctioned from the patient's abdomen and then transferred into devolumized areas of the face. The stem cell facelift differs from fat-grafting procedures of years past because the fat is harvested and injected with special cannulas (tubes) to ensure survival of the grafted tissue. Fat cells are extremely fragile, and the main goal is to make sure they survive once transplanted. Once harvested, the fat is processed to maximize the amount of adult stem cells present in the fat that is transplanted. An adult stem cell is an undifferentiated (has no distinguishing features) cell that can renew itself and can differentiate to yield some or all of the major specialized cell types of a tissue or organ. The primary roles of adult stem cells in a living organism are to maintain and repair the tissue in which they are found.

Adult stem cells are now known to be a source for producing other hormone-like substances and growth factors to enhance both skin quality and the underlying subcutaneous fatty tissues of the cheeks, mid-face, and skin in general.

Stem cell facelifts add fat back to the drooped cheeks, jawline, and smile and marionette lines. The face refills and lifts (like a saggy

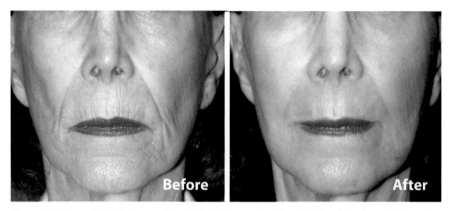

Figure 15. Patient who had a "stem cell facelift" with fat transferred to the deflated cheeks to lift them along the jawline; fat transfers were also used in the folds around the mouth to lift jowling and in the hollows in the temple that occur with advancing age. The face looks rejuvenated and softer.

deflated balloon lifts as it is reinflated), creating the heart-shaped face of youth instead of the square-shape face of middle age. Additionally, fat can be injected into the deep circles under the eyes, creating the appearance of a lower eyelids lift without surgery. Fat is globular and thick and cannot be injected into fine surface lines as it would make them look lumpy. The sites we more specifically place these injections are discussed in chapter 5.

The stem cell facelift procedure itself, which is usually done on an outpatient basis, is also relatively straightforward: the fat is harvested under local anesthesia using suction and aspiration with a needle. The fat is then processed to prepare for injection. Lastly, the fat is injected under local anesthesia in the desired area.

Recovery time takes about a week. At the end of this time, light makeup can be applied. The stem cell facelift may eliminate the need for ongoing facial filler injections like Restylane, Juvederm, and the other hyaluronic acid fillers. Sometimes the procedure needs to be repeated more than once because the fat and adult stem cells only partially "take" in the face where they are injected. On average, 33 percent of patients will require more than one treatment session. Once the fat grafting has taken, the results usually last three to five years before a repeat treatment or other intervention would be required.

For those with more-advanced facial drooping and aging, a facelift or eyelid lift may be necessary. Simply doing a fat transfer on a person in their forties and early fifties can rejuvenate their face without lifting it, but in the mid-fifties into the sixties, filling alone causes the face to take on a more amorphous, overfilled, and round appearance. This can look altered or unnatural. We see this in many celebrities, as discussed in chapter 2.

Although there is no exact age when the face needs to be supported by a lifting procedure, the most common age that I consult with women is when they are three years postmenopausal. In America, this is on average 53.8 years old. At this time of life, without estrogen stimulation of the face, the quality of the skin changes significantly

> During a stem cell facelift, fat is processed to maximize the amount of adult stem cells present in the fat that is transplanted. Adult stem cells are now known to be a source for producing growth factors to enhance both skin quality and the underlying subcutaneous fatty tissues of the cheeks, the mid-face, and skin in general.

and the facial muscles loosen more in 3 years than in the prior 50. In older faces it is not enough to simply fill the face because the facial tissues cannot support the additional volume when they have become too loose.

Although a standard facelift surgery repositions drooped fat (like the jowls) into areas of volume loss, it is often necessary to combine a facelift with a fat transfer. Older faces can lose so much volume that lifting the cheeks is not sufficient, and volume needs to be added back into the cheeks.

The Vampire Facelift

The Vampire Facelift uses an injectable product called Selphyl. It works the same way a liquid facelift or stem cell facelift works, except it uses Selphyl. It is done by drawing a patient's blood and separating the platelets from the red blood cells. The separated platelets are then mixed with a fibrin mixture, creating a gel that is injected into the area to be augmented. Surgeons overfill the area by 20 percent, so a patient can see an approximation of the final results. The excess fill will be gone in about a day. Several weeks after the blood injection facelift, the fibrin matrix builds up and the final result appears. I find that patients like the idea that Selphyl uses their own blood's natural resources to treat wrinkles.

Selphyl claims that the Vampire Facelift lasts about fifteen months. Although I have never performed this procedure, colleagues performing the treatment tell me the procedure's longevity is similar to the length of most hyaluronic acid fillers or even shorter. The cost of a Sephyl injection is more than that of an equivalent volume of

> **If you are very thin with minimal body fat, you may not be a good candidate for fat transfer. I tend to use Radiesse and Sculptra Aesthetic for volumizing in patients with thin faces and not enough fat to transplant.**

hyaluronic acid filler. To my mind, it can, therefore, be more expensive than a hyaluronic acid filler injection session without an additional benefit of longevity.

I have spoken with dozens of patients who have had the treatment performed elsewhere who say the same thing about its longevity. There is only one clinical trial published in the medical literature that discusses the safety of Selphyl, and it doesn't mention how long its effect actually lasts. I do believe it to be a safe treatment that works, but I would be wary of the company's claim that it lasts fifteen months until more definitive studies prove that it lasts this long.

References

Sclafani, A.P. 2011. Safety, efficacy, and utility of platelet-rich fibrin matrix in facial plastic surgery. *Archives of Facial Plastic Surgery.* Jul-Aug; 13(4): 247-251.

Tabit, C.J., G.C. Slack, K. Fan, et al. 2011. fat grafting versus adipose-derived stem cell therapy: distinguishing indications, techniques, and outcomes. *Aesthetic Plastic Surgery.* Nov 9.

Yeh, C.C., E. F. Williams, 3rd. 2001. Long-term results of autologous periorbital lipotransfer. *Archives of Facial Plastic Surgery.* Jul-Aug; 13(4): 252-258.

7 Skin Rejuvenation with Laser and Energy-Based System Treatments

The skin can age at a normal chronological rate, in which case you will look as old as you are. Your skin can age at an accelerated rate, in which case you will tend to look older than your chronological age). If your skin ages at a decreased rate, you may look younger than you really are.

If you'd like to erase signs of aging, there are literally hundreds of lasers and light-based devices on the market today, and new ones are being developed.

When people hear the word "laser," they automatically have high expectations. A laser is a high-energy light beam that is extremely focused and capable of delivering high amounts of energy to a small area. These devices have the ability to specifically target a particular color or molecule. Each device targets different molecules, such as the red hemoglobin found in blood vessels or the brown found in freckles. To remove skin that is sun-damaged and wrinkled, lasers that are absorbed by water might be utilized to vaporize the damaged layers.

Other light sources, such as intense pulsed lights, are multitasking devices that are capable of treating many different skin problems. However, they are not technically lasers. Lasers of different colors, called frequencies, and energy levels can treat a variety of skin problems including: unwanted hair, acne, port wine stains, scars, psoriasis, skin cancers, tattoos, blood vessels, wrinkles, laxity of the skin, freckles, scars, and stretch marks. To optimize treatment, you may need a combination of several lasers.

Intense Pulsed Light Therapy (IPL)

The most popular energy-based systems are intense pulsed light or IPL devices. Intense pulsed light (IPL) is exactly what it sounds like:

Ten Signs of Aging Skin

- uneven complexion
- enlarged pores
- broken capillaries
- dry, rough patches
- loss of radiance
- pigmentation
- lines and wrinkles
- sagging skin
- sallow appearance
- skin growths

intense light of all wavelengths. It differs from a laser, which utilizes coherent light of a single color (wavelength). Different wavelengths (colors) of light interact with the skin in different ways. To treat red discolorations of the skin (such as telangiectasias or rosacea), light absorbed by the color of hemoglobin (found within the blood vessels) is the best choice. Freckles, brown spots, and unwanted hair may all be treated with light of a particular color.

To accomplish specific goals, most intense pulsed lights have different hand pieces that emit different colors of light. Intense pulsed light is also helpful for treating acne and actinic keratoses or precancerous lesions. IPL is also often combined with other treatments such as BOTOX Cosmetic, microdermabrasion, and peels. IPL has also been helpful in treating superficial age spots on the face and hands, as well as for the treatment of neck discoloration.

Typical IPL treatments are performed every three to six weeks and a series of four to six treatments is recommended. Minor discomfort— comparable to a rubber band snapping on your skin—is typical for treatment with IPL. Following a treatment, dark spots may appear darker as they lift through the skin and migrate off. Red lesions may appear slightly bruised. Following IPL treatments, you should expect a more even tone and texture. Treatments for acne and rosacea produce gradual improvements over the span of a few months. IPL is considered a workhorse because it treats many skin conditions with little or no downtime.

Sometimes more treatments than expected are necessary, possibly up to eight to ten treatments, depending upon how resistant the condition is. These additional treatments can be frustrating to both the patient and the doctor. After full treatment, it is often necessary to have one or two treatments a year to prevent recurrence of the skin's textural and color changes. Avoiding the sun and using sunblocks as described in chapter 3 are essential to prevent rapid return of the same issues over the course of a few months, especially after many months of IPL treatments.

Skin Resurfacing

Since the days of ancient Egypt, people have been using resurfacing methods to rejuvenate skin. The original chemical peel was lactic acid, an active ingredient of sour milk that was used topically by the nobles as part of an ancient skin-rejuvenation regimen. In the Middle Ages, old wine with tartaric acid as its active ingredient was used for the

> Do not have any skin-resurfacing treatments (peels, microdermabrasion, IPL, lasers) if you have a recent tan or have taken Accutane or isotretinoin (a potent drug for cystic acne) for the past six months as it can cause skin discoloration or scarring.

same purpose. Today, these historical peeling solutions are known to contain alpha hydroxy acids (AHAs), which are the active ingredients responsible for the skin exfoliation.

Physicians use a grading scale for wrinkles called the Glogau Scale, created by Dr. Richard Glogau. The rating on this scale will often dictate the treatment, as I will discuss later. The Glogau skin-aging classification scale is as follows:

- Glogau 1—Mild (age 28–35 years)—minimal to no discoloration or wrinkling, no keratoses (skin overgrowths), generally no need for foundation or makeup

- Glogau 2—Moderate (age 35–50 years)—wrinkling as skin moves, slight lines near the eyes and mouth, usually a need for some foundation

- Glogau 3—Advanced (age 50–60 years)—visible wrinkles all the time, noticeable discolorations, visible keratoses, generally a need for heavy foundation

- Glogau 4—Severe (age 65–70 years)—severe wrinkling throughout, gravitational and dynamic forces affecting skin, yellow or gray color to skin, makeup not usable because it cakes and cracks

Resurfacing procedures can be identified along a ladder of aggressivity, from superficial treatments, to medium-depth treatment, to deep treatments. The difference among these procedures has to do with the layer of the skin they remove: Superficial treatments generally remove and resurface the epidermis, or top layer of the skin; medium-depth treatments get down to the medium depth (half thickness) of the dermis; and deep treatments get down into the deeper two-thirds of the dermis. The appropriate treatment is based on the depth of the wrinkle, or the layer of the skin the crevice extends into.

The three classifications of resurfacing procedures are chemical peels, laser resurfacing, and dermabrasion. The major difference among these treatments is that chemical energy is used to polish the skin in a chemical peel, light/heat energy is used with lasers, and mechanical (sandpaper-like) energy is used with dermabrasion.

> Your skin color dictates what skin resurfacing treatments are safe. Not everyone is a candidate for every resurfacing procedure. Patients with darker skin are at risk for changes in their skin color with more-aggressive treatments: either the skin can lighten (hypopigment) or darken (hyperpigment).

Your skin color dictates what treatments are safe. Not everyone is a candidate for every resurfacing procedure. Patients with darker skin are at risk for changes in their skin color with more aggressive treatments. Either the skin can lighten (hypopigment) or darken (hyperpigment). Yes, as you already guessed, physicians have a classification for the darkness of skin, and it is called the Fitzpatrick Scale. This classification denotes six different skin types, skin colors, and reactions to sun exposure.

- Type I (very white or freckled)—always burn
- Type II (white)—usually burn
- Type III (white to olive)—sometimes burn
- Type IV (brown)—rarely burn
- Type V (dark brown)—very rarely burn
- Type VI (black)—never burn

People with Type IV skin or greater generally are at a higher risk for pigmentary disturbance after medium and deep resurfacing procedures. They are often better off staying with more superficial treatments or fractional laser resurfacing as will be described later in this chapter.

Superficial Skin Resurfacing and Microdermabrasion

Superficial resurfacing can be accomplished by all three methods and has the advantage of little or no downtime. These procedures can be done at lunchtime and one can return to work after a treatment. There can be some mild redness and irritation associated with them for a day or two, but there are no raw surfaces to heal. These treatments are usually performed repeatedly over a short period of time.

For example, a chemical peel is performed weekly for three months. The theory is that repeated resurfacing will not only remove the dead layers of cells from the epidermis, tighten pores, and soften fine lines and wrinkles, but also will stimulate collagen production in the dermis and tighten the surface. A chemical peel will not treat deeper skin lines like "lipstick bleed lines" or deeper forehead lines and crow's feet because they do not penetrate deep enough into the skin. These treatments are generally safe for patients with dark skin types.

Alpha (AHA) and Beta (BHA) Hydroxy Acid Chemical Peels

These acids are derived from fruit, milk, and other natural sources. The most common of these is glycolic acid, which is derived from sugarcane. They are very effective at turning over the skin's dead surface layer, stimulating collagen production, and smoothing the skin surface.

Microdermabrasion

This technique uses mechanical energy, with small crystals sprayed at the skin surface under pressure. A vacuum sucks the dead skin cells and crystals. The pressure can be increased with repeated treatments to affect a better result. This treatment, like all of its class, is "wash and wear"—there is no downtime. Microdermabrasion is very different from its distant relative which I call "macrodermabrasion;" this procedure involves using a rotating abrasive brush that reaches the medium and deep layers of the skin.

"Light Touch" Lasers

These lasers are nonablative; this means they do not melt the skin away with light and heat energy like their more aggressive counterparts which I discuss later in this chapter. These laser types (Nd:YAG, alexandrite, and pulsed dye) will reorganize the collagen in the dermal

65

layers of the skin, tighten it, and give it a better texture. A cool-touch version is available that uses a cooling tip to minimize the discomfort during treatment.

Medium-Depth Resurfacing, Lasers, and Skin Peels

Medium-depth resurfacing procedures traditionally include trichloroacetic acid (TCA) peels and laser resurfacing. There is a new classification of medium-depth lasers that are called fractional lasers, which I describe below. These procedures can get rid of the majority of the fine wrinkles in the skin completely, unlike superficial resurfacing that results in these lines only becoming softer. I often tell patients that medium-depth procedures will get rid of about 60 percent of the lines. Since these procedures resurface down to the mid-dermal layer, they can remove the deeper wrinkles while causing the skin to tighten with the production of more collagen.

Medium-depth resurfacing procedures have a greater risk of complications than the superficial peels but are extremely safe when used on the correct skin type by a skilled plastic surgeon or dermatologist. Patients with Fitzpatrick Class IV skin (darker complexions that tan easily) and higher can experience pigmentary changes in the skin, including lightening and darkening of different areas, so they are generally not good candidates. Scarring is another possible adverse outcome, but with the appropriate laser energy settings, and at the appropriate depths of peeling, the risks are extremely low.

Unlike superficial resurfacing treatments, these procedures can be painful when performed while you're awake. Local anesthetic injections to numb the skin surface, or "twilight" anesthesia, which makes you doze, are the ways that I keep patients comfortable.

All deeper resurfacing procedures require that you take anti-herpes simplex virus treatment before and during the recovery phase because there is a risk of the chicken pox virus reactivating and causing ulcers. These can cause scarring while healing. As always, an ounce of prevention is worth a pound of cure.

Trichloroacetic Acid (TCA) Peels

TCA peels can be administered in 20 percent, 30 percent, 35 percent, and 40 percent levels, and as the percentage increases the depth of the peel increases. At lower concentrations it can be applied with the use of a local anesthetic to numb the skin; with higher concentrations, I believe it is better to have a "twilight" anesthesia

66

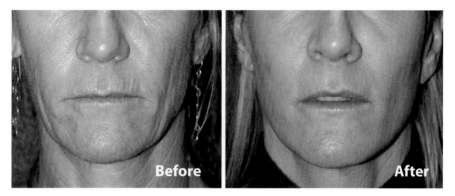

Figure 16. Patient who had a fractional CO2 laser skin resurfacing to reduce facial wrinkles and lipstick bleed lines around the mouth.

where you are not awake, but you are not under the effects of general anesthesia. This is the type of anesthesia you might get in a dentist's office or during a colonoscopy. After a TCA peel is applied, there is no pain or burning past the application of the solution. Moisturizing ointments are applied for the ensuing week, and after about four days the dead skin surface peels off, almost like the way old paint flakes off a wall. One week after the procedure, all the skin has peeled and this leaves very smooth, new pink skin underneath that almost looks like you have a sunburn. This pinkness fades during the ensuing three weeks, but camouflaging makeup can be applied one week after a peel.

Carbon Dioxide (CO2) and Erbium:YAG Laser Resurfacing

Unlike the superficial light-touch lasers, these are ablative lasers that remove the skin layers by vaporizing or melting the skin. Removal of the medium depth of skin with a laser encourages the growth of healthy new cells. The thermal effect of the CO_2 laser on collagen causes the skin to tighten a little more than with a TCA peel. The Erbium:YAG laser is most commonly used for fine lines and wrinkles. It is a less-aggressive laser than the CO_2 laser and uses a different wavelength of light that causes less thermal injury. The heat energy causes collagen contraction and new collagen formation in the dermal layers of the skin.

The improvement seen in deeper wrinkles with Erbium:YAG is not as good as with the CO_2 laser, even at the same depth of penetration. The advantage to the Erbium:YAG laser over the CO_2 laser is its lower risk of scarring and lightening of the skin's color, which has been reported in some medical literature to happen in as high as 7 percent of patients. After all medium-depth laser resurfacing, an occlusive dressing is applied and not removed for five days, allowing the skin to regenerate and heal over the surface. As with medium-depth chemical peels, all raw surfaces are healed over at seven days, and the skin remains pink for the ensuing three weeks.

Deep Skin Resurfacing

The most aggressive way to resurface the skin is with a phenol peel or macrodermabrasion. Since this procedure resurfaces to the deep dermal layer, called the reticular dermis, it can remove the deepest wrinkles while causing the skin to tighten with the production of more collagen. These resurfacing methods are used on patients classified as *severe* or Class 4 on the Glogau Scale noted above. Due to the aggressivity of deep resurfacing, there are greater risks of scarring and hypopigmentation (skin whitening).

Have you ever noticed how older Hollywood celebrities' skin can almost appear translucent and pale, yet line free? This is the appearance of an individual that has had multiple deep resurfacings. The initial healing phase for these procedures is much longer than for medium-depth resurfacing, taking approximately two weeks, and the pink tone to the skin can last up to three months.

Phenol Peels

Phenol produces the most dramatic results and is the most effective peeling agent currently used. The phenol produces a new zone of collagen that is thicker than that produced by laser or macrodemabrasion. The toxicity of phenol may be significant and the procedure should be performed only by a physician who regularly performs this aggressive treatment. Phenol is absorbed through the skin, metabolized by the liver, and subsequently excreted by the kidneys. Overdoses may injure the liver and kidney and may lead to heart problems. For this reason, phenol peels should always be performed in an operating room, with a board-certified anesthesiologist present.

Macrodermabrasion

This method is much different from microdermabrasion which is more like a loofah sponge for the skin, exfoliating and removing only the surface layer (epidermis) of the skin. Unlike a chemical peel that uses chemical energy, and a laser resurfacing that uses heat energy, dermabrasion is the process of mechanically removing the damaged layers of skin. In a lot of ways, a macrodermabraded area is no different from a scraped knee. Usually a rotating brush or diamond wheel is used to penetrate into the depth of the skin in a graduated fashion. Because it is extremely dependent on the skill of the surgeon, this process can be viewed almost as an art, with the physician sculpting the skin. Macrodermabrasion is wonderful for the deeper lines, especially those that radiate around the lips, the so-called lipstick bleed lines. The healing phase is usually two weeks. An occlusive dressing is worn as in laser resurfacing; however, the skin surface tends to weep, draining fluid for the first few days.

Fractional Laser Devices

Until the advent of fractional laser devices, two varieties of laser treatment had been available for cosmetic enhancement: ablative (CO_2 and Erbium:YAG) and nonablative (IPL), as described above. Ablative, which literally means to vaporize at a very high temperature, is very effective at destroying unwanted tissue but has significant side effects and requires a lengthy healing period. Nonablative, on the other hand, has very few side effects and requires almost no healing time but involves numerous treatments over many months to achieve only modest results.

Throughout the past few years, the concept of fractional laser skin resurfacing has evolved. With fractional skin rejuvenation, an Erbium:YAG laser beam is broken up or fractionated into many small microbeams which are separated so that when they strike the skin surface small areas of the skin between the beams are not hit by the laser and are left intact. The small areas treated by the fractional microbeams, called micro treatment zones, create new collagen to replace collagen damaged by aging and sun exposure. Damage to collagen in the skin is a cause of skin wrinkles.

The new collagen produced by the laser injury "plumps" skin wrinkles. The intact skin between the micro treatment zones allows for much more rapid healing—twenty-four to forty-eight hours of some skin redness and swelling as opposed to two to three weeks of open skin wounds, weeping, and crusting of the skin for the older CO_2 laser and deeper peels, and enough pigment cells are left intact so that hypopigmentation does not occur. The Erbium:YAG fractional laser usually requires three to five treatments to get good results with skin wrinkles.

The wrinkle removal achieved by ablative CO_2 resurfacing is more significant because ablation removes damaged, aged skin as well as heats the deeper skin layers to promote new collagen production. But with this comes the increased risk of hypopigmentation or loss of pigment and "whitening" of the skin and scarring.

To decrease the risks of fully ablative CO_2, several new fractional CO_2 ablative lasers have been developed which have the benefits of fractional treatments, less downtime, fewer complications, as well as ablative skin resurfacing, better wrinkle removal, and facial rejuvenation. Figure 17 shows how this new technology works in comparison to previous laser methods.

Another benefit of fractional skin rejuvenation is that, unlike older ablative laser resurfacing techniques, the new fractional skin rejuvenation lasers appear to be safe to use on darker Asian and African-American skin. This will make the latest skin-rejuvenation techniques available to millions of people with dark skin, Fitzpatrick Scale Type IV and above, who could not be safely treated with previous skin-rejuvenation techniques.

Skin Tightening

Radiofrequency-Based Systems

Radiofrequency waves can be delivered to the deep layers of the skin (the dermis layers) which stimulates collagen production while leaving the skin's surface (the epidermis) relatively untouched. Collagen fibers, which are essential for firm, youthful-looking skin, tend to degenerate as we age, mainly because of overexposure to the sun. In addition to stimulating new collagen, radiofrequency treatment also causes some contraction of the skin, thus tightening it. Although you'll notice the treatment's tightening effects immediately, the more significant improvements will occur gradually over a period of several weeks or months as the new collagen forms.

There are a number of radiofrequency devices on the market today, including ones that have one pole, called monopolar, delivering the radiofrequency waves to the skin, and others with two poles, called bipolar. Some of the most common devices are Thermage, Titan, and Aluma.

My experience with radiofrequency tightening of the skin is that the results are not very predictable. It works well (15 percent improvement) in some patients but not well in others. I own a

Ablative Resurfacing (CO2 & 2.94 Erb:YAG)	Non-Ablative Fractional Resurfacing (Erbium: YAG) 600-1,000 microns	Ablative Fractional Resurfacing CO2 600-1,000 microns

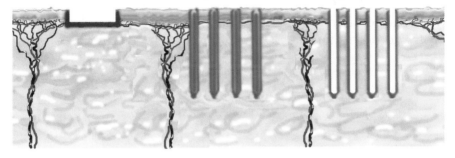

Figure 17. The diagram above shows the progression of laser skin rejuvenation technology from the older fully ablative CO² (left) to the newest fractional ablative lasers (right).

radiofrequency device but no longer use it due to the more predictable and better results I have seen with the ultrasonic energy device that I will discuss next.

Ultrasonic Energy

Ultherapy is the first and only ultrasound energy-based device for aesthetics cleared by the FDA with a noninvasive "lift" indication for the neck, face, and eyebrows. Ultrasound is sound at frequencies higher than those detected by human hearing (at least 18 kilohertz or 18,000 cycles per second). Unlike radiofrequency treatments, as described above, and lasers that typically involve improving superficial layers of the skin, Ultherapy addresses the deep skin layers and the foundational layer addressed in cosmetic surgery that lends support to the skin. This layer in the face is called the SMAS (superficial muscular aponeurotic system) and in the neck is called the platysma.

With ultrasound, we can bypass the upper layers of the skin and deliver the *right* amount of energy at the *right* depths to contract and then ultimately lift the SMAS and platysma. As a result, there is no damage on the surface of the skin so there is no downtime with this therapy. Ultrasound triggers the body's natural response mechanism, which is to rejuvenate tired collagen and supplement it with fresh, new collagen. Collagen is the protein latticework that provides structure to the skin and to the deep supportive connective tissue and muscles below the skin. Upon treatment, the regenerative process is initiated, but the full effect

71

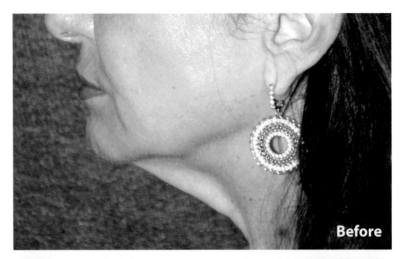

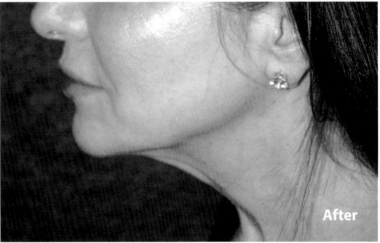

Figure 18. Patient who had Ultherapy to tighten the jawline and neck. Notice an approximately 30 percent tightening effect without surgery.

will build gradually over the course of two to three months.

You may immediately experience a slight lifting and toning and get a tighter, firmer feel. After the first month, you may experience slight lifting and toning, a tighter, firmer feel and a smoother texture. When you start your second and third months you may experience better-fitting skin, reduced sagging, "openness" around the eyes, a sleeker jawline, and improved contour under the chin. This treatment takes approximately one hour and can be painful for patients, so we administer ibuprofen before treatment to minimize discomfort.

While Ultherapy does not duplicate the results of surgery, it is an inviting alternative for those who are not ready for surgery but want meaningful results. The Ultherapy appeal is also great for patients with beginning signs of skin laxity. Skin laxity commonly first occurs on the forehead, which leads to brow descent, excess skin/hooding on the lids, and a less open-eyed appearance. Cheek and neck tissue laxity can lead to flattening of the mid-cheek, nasolabial folds, marionette lines on the chin, downturned mouth, loss of jawline angularity, jowls, and sagging under the chin.

Young patients wanting to stay ahead of the aging process, trendsetters wanting the latest innovation, and patients wanting to complement other procedures are also good candidates for Ultherapy. Factors affecting treatment response include skin laxity (amount of excess, loose skin on the face or neck), volume (degree and distribution of fat), skin quality (extent of lines, wrinkles, crepey skin, and/or sun damage), age (twenties/thirties, forties to sixties, seventies and up), and lifestyle/health (smoker, nature of health issues).

The results of this treatment are also dependent upon facial structure. Improvements range from 10 to 35 percent tightening in my experience. Better results occur in patients with thin skin, a defined jawline, strong cheek and chin structure, and less facial fat. Patients with a chubby face, thick skin, weak skeletal structure, and a very heavy face tend to have less improvement. In these cases, sometimes more than one treatment of Ultherapy is required or surgery is recommended.

I will often combine the Utherapy sessions with Sculptra Aesthetic injections; the synergistic effects of both treatments are amazing and create what I call a "nonsurgical facelift." Sculptra Aesthetic helps to add the volume back to the face that has deflated with age. Ultherapy tightens but does not replenish the facial volume we lose as we age. An older face will show a loss of the fullness of the cheeks, temples, lips, and area around the mouth and will show fat loss under the eyes which creates a hollow effect. Where there used to be light, now there are shadows. By replacing the volume loss, you reverse the creation of shadow and restore the reflection of light and the appearance of youth, energy, and vibrancy. This volume replacement fills the skin so that it is lifted by the formation of your body's own collagen—collagen that was created in surrounding the microscopic particles that make up Sculptra Aesthetic.

References

Alexiades-Armenaka, M., D. Sarnoff, R. Gotkin, N. Sadick. 2011. Multi-center clinical study and review of fractional ablative CO_2 laser resurfacing for the treatment of rhytides, photoaging, scars and striae. *Journal of Drugs of Dermatology.* Apr; 10(4): 352-362.

Bass, L.S. 2005. Rejuvenation of the aging face using Fraxel laser treatment. *Aesthetic Surgery Journal.* May-Jun; 25(3): 307-309.

Fritz, M., J.T. Counters, B.D. Zelickson. 2004. Radiofrequency treatment for middle and lower face laxity. *Archives of Facial Plastic Surgery.* 2004; 6(6): 370-373.

Lee, H.S., W.S. Jang, Y.J. Cha, et al. 2012. Multiple-pass ultrasound tightening of skin laxity of the lower face and neck. *Dermatologic Surgery.* Jan; 38(1): 20-27.

Tanzi, E.L., and T.S. Alster. 2003. Single-pass carbon dioxide versus multiple-pass Er:YAG laser skin resurfacing: A comparison of postoperative wound healing and side-effect rates. *Dermatologic Surgery.* Jan; 29(1): 80-84.

8 State-of-the-Art Hair Restoration

Hair loss may come as a surprise, but it is no mystery. As we age, the rate of hair growth slows. The most common cause of thinning hair is heredity, and this trait can be passed down from either your mother's or your father's side of the family. You may notice areas of hair that no longer need cutting and where the hairs are getting shorter and finer. It is important to know that finding hairs in your tub, sink, or brush is not necessarily a sign of thinning hair. This could indicate a temporary hair-loss condition. It is natural for hair to go through a constant cycle of growth and resting or dormancy.

If you are not on your way to balding, your hair will grow back just as strong. If you are balding, your hair will grow back finer and will not grow as long before falling out again. What you see in the mirror over a longer period is the best monitor of early signs of thinning. Both men and women suffer hair loss, but patterns may be different in women than in men.

It is estimated that 35 million men in the United States are affected by male pattern baldness or *androgenetic alopecia.* "Andro" refers to the androgens (testosterone, dihydrotestosterone) necessary to produce male-pattern hair loss (MPHL). "Genetic" refers to the inherited gene necessary for MPHL to occur. In men who develop male pattern baldness, the hair loss may begin any time after puberty when blood levels of androgens rise.

The first change is usually recession in the temporal areas, which is seen in 96 percent of mature Caucasian males, including those men not destined to progress to further hair loss. Later, the frontal hairline recedes, resulting ultimately in a classic "horseshoe" fringe of hair and a bald crown and frontal hairline. Whether this happens in the twenties, thirties, forties, fifties, or beyond is related to genetic factors.

Female pattern baldness is usually different from that of male pattern baldness. The hair thins all over the head, but the frontal hairline is maintained. There may be a moderate loss of hair on the crown, but this rarely progresses to total or near baldness as it may in men.

Every person who desires to have his or her baldness or hair loss corrected must be treated on an individual basis. Choosing hair restoration surgery is a major decision for most people and will permanently change their appearance to a more youthful look. Hair transplant surgery will restore hair that will grow naturally and require styling and haircuts, just like the hair of persons who do not suffer from hair loss.

How Hair Is Transplanted: Microfollicular Unit Grafting

The essence of these procedures is that the hair is transplanted into the balding area as individual follicular units, so that it will look totally natural and be undetectable as a hair transplant. With hair transplant procedures, hair is "harvested" or taken from areas of the head where growth is not affected by balding and is transplanted into the balding areas. With modern techniques, very small hair grafts, called individual follicular units, are used so that the hairline and hair will look natural. If you look closely under magnification at how hair naturally grows, you can see that hair grows in clusters of one, two, three, and sometimes four hairs. These naturally occurring groups of hair are called "follicular hair units."

We can transfer these follicles to be placed closer together to create a dense-looking head of hair. Micrografting is a delicate and time-consuming process. Each follicular hair unit has to be kept intact and trimmed under a microscope to create the ultimate micrograft. The end result is a hair transplant that can be undetectable.

Older technology using "plugs" with groups of twenty or more hairs made hair transplantation very obvious, almost making the hair appear like the hair coming out of the scalp of a child's doll, thus the reference to hair plugs that look like "doll's hair."

I am now able to transplant up to 2,500 grafts in what I call a megasession. Follicular unit grafts require more time, skill, and a dedicated, well-trained staff compared to the mini/micrografts that were previously performed. This technique may entail five assistants working with microscopes for many hours or the whole day. Depending

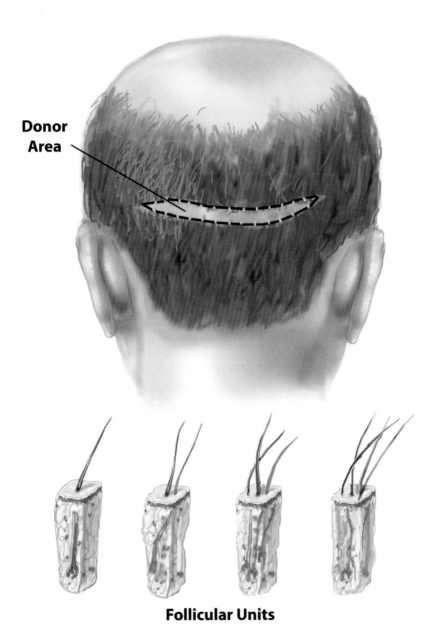

Donor Area

Follicular Units

Figure 19. Hair transplants are harvested from a donor area on the back of the head. Hair grows out of the scalp with one, two, three, or four hairs coming out of each follicle. These follicular units are transplanted separately to create natural looking hairlines.

upon the degree of balding, and the degree of hair density desired, patients may require up to two or three megasessions. In female pattern baldness, the goal is to create more hair density over large areas of the scalp, so multiple megasessions are required.

There are two techniques that differ in the way the hair is harvested (removed) from the donor area in the back of the scalp: follicular unit transplantation (FUT) and follicular unit extraction (FUE).

Follicular Unit Transplantation

In follicular unit transplantation, a thin strip of hair is taken from the back and/or sides of the scalp, and the area where the strip was taken from is sewn closed. The hair is removed in a single, thin strip and then, with the use of microscopes, is dissected into individual follicular units. The hair from above the incision covers the area so that it is not visible. The donor strip is placed under a series of special dissecting microscopes where the individual follicular units, of one to four hairs each, are carefully dissected into tiny grafts. These grafts are stored in a special holding solution and refrigerated while awaiting placement.

The recipient sites (tiny incisions) are made in the bald or thinning areas of the scalp using a fine needle-size instrument. Once the recipient sites are made, the follicular unit grafts are carefully inserted into the scalp. The one-hair grafts are placed at the hairline, the two-hair grafts immediately behind them, and the larger three- and four-hair units are placed in the central forelock area. The recipient site sizes are matched to the different-size follicular unit grafts to facilitate healing and maximize the growth of the transplanted follicles.

Follicular Unit Extraction

In follicular unit extraction (FUE), a relatively large area in the back and sides of the scalp is shaved to approximately one millimeter in length. Instead of removing a single strip, as in FUT, a tiny circular incision is made around each follicular unit. The follicular units are removed directly from the back and sides of the scalp using a robotic device. The follicular units are then extracted, one by one, directly from the scalp. These grafts are stored in a special holding solution and refrigerated while awaiting placement in the bald or thinning scalp (the recipient area). The tiny wounds are left open to heal on their own.

As in FUT, recipient sites (tiny incisions) are made in the bald or thinning areas of the scalp using a fine needle-size instrument. The follicular unit grafts are then placed into these sites.

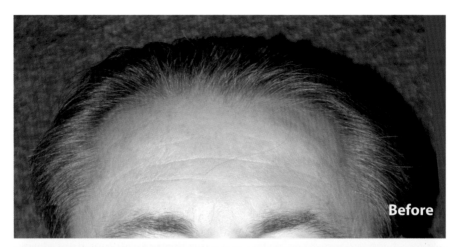

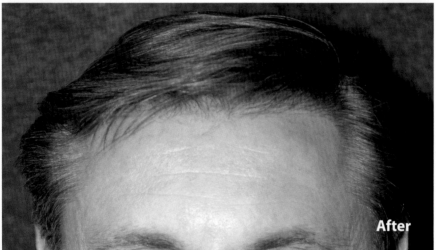

Figure 20. Follicular unit hair transplantation creates a youthful-looking hairline.

Shaping the Hairline

The artistry in hair transplantation comes in how the surgeon blends as well as shapes the hairline. If the hairline is constructed like a straight edge, it will appear artificial. The hairline needs to have a natural wave, similar to that of your original hairline. Additionally, the hairline should not be placed too low. In patients with more severe baldness, more than one hair transplant session will be required to restore the hairline. The first few transplant sessions are dedicated to the front of the hairline above the forehead. This frames the face which is the aesthetic priority in hair transplantation. Once this is accomplished, later hair transplant sessions are focused on a balding crown. Those with just balding in the crown of the scalp can just have just that area treated.

Most hair restoration procedures are performed under local anesthesia which means no "general" anesthesia and therefore a quick recovery that will not affect your ability to go back to work. Hair transplant sessions that use thousands of follicular unit grafts may take a whole day; however, the time goes by quickly. During the procedure, patients rest comfortably and can watch TV or a movie, take a nap, or chat with the staff.

The misperceptions that people may have of hair transplantation— that patients leave the office with their heads wrapped in bandages and have significant bleeding and pain—are leftover images from the outdated plug techniques. With modern follicular unit hair transplants, patients leave the office with only a hat and headband and are able to shower and shampoo their hair the day after the hair restoration surgery.

References

Onda, M., H.H. Igawa, K. Inoue, et al. 2008. Novel technique of follicular unit extraction hair transplantation with a powered punching device. *Dermatologic Surgery*. Dec; 34(12): 1683-1688.

Tan Baser, N., B. Cigsar, U. Balci Akbuga, et al. 2006. Follicular unit transplantation for male-pattern hair loss: Evaluation of 120 patients. *Journal of Plastic Reconstructive Aesthetic Surgery*. 59(11): 1162-1169.

PART III.

My Surgical Approach

9 Anesthesia: Local or General?

Every day in my practice I am asked by patients whether their surgery can be performed without general anesthesia. General anesthesia involves being paralyzed during surgery with medications administered by an anesthesiologist, receiving a breathing tube, and breathing anesthetic gas. Patients are concerned about the risks involved with having general anesthesia as it puts a significant amount of strain on the body. Other patients have experienced days of feeling ill with nausea, headaches, and weakness after general anesthesia and want to avoid it at all costs.

My answer to them is that we rarely use general anesthesia in my practice when performing facial plastic surgery. In fact, I prefer not to use it unless it is necessary because the patient has some other medical condition that requires it. General anesthetic drugs and gases cause major physiologic changes in the body; they cause blood vessels to dilate, increasing how much you bleed during surgery. This causes bruising and swelling, which increases recovery time. Additionally, general anesthesia can induce vomiting which can lead to further trauma and torn sutures for some patients.

Local Anesthesia

When I perform surgery on patients, I give them different options for their anesthesia, because it is not a one-size-fits-all approach. I perform surgery either under a local anesthesia, which means the patient is wide awake and has surgery after numbing shots are administered, or under a twilight anesthesia given through an IV (no anesthesia gas is given) so the patient is asleep and not aware. In my practice only 30 percent of my patients do surgery wide awake under a local anesthetic; 70 percent of patients have a twilight anesthetic where they are asleep for the surgery, but in *no* case are they under general anesthesia.

Facelifts, rhinoplasties ("nose jobs"), eyelid lifts, lip augmentaton surgery, chin and cheek augmentation, and many other procedures can easily and safely be performed under local anesthesia. This means being given a minor sedative like Valium in a pill form to relax you, then novocaine-like local shots (similar to the ones you would get at

> Facelifts, rhinoplasties ("nose jobs"), eyelid lifts, lip augmentation surgery, chin and cheek augmentation, and many other procedures can easily and safely be performed under local anesthesia without general anesthesia.

the dentist) to numb the part of the face having surgery. We use the drugs Lidocaine and Marcaine because they last longer and are more effective than novocaine. The shots can be painful and multiple shots need to be administered, but we use a tiny needle that spreads the medicine slowly to minimize discomfort. Because of this discomfort, I do not suggest this procedure for those who are afraid of needles or have a very low pain threshold. The value in local anesthesia is that it decreases the amount of bleeding during surgery when compared to general anesthesia, and therefore bruising and postoperative recovery is lessened. Also, because the surgeon gives the shots to numb the face, you do not have to pay for an anesthesiologist to administer anesthesia so there are additional cost savings.

We also employ music therapy prior to injections and during the local anesthesia surgery. It has been shown that playing relaxing music that a patient prefers helps lower patient's blood pressure during surgery. This limits bleeding and, therefore, minimizes bruising.

Twilight Sedation

For patients who do not want to be awake and aware during surgery, we perform a twilight anesthesia. This medication is like an intravenous Valium, but as soon as the medicine is turned off, you wake up in a few minutes without any nausea, headache or hangover from general anesthesia gas. Twilight anesthesia also reduces bruising compared to the effect of general anesthesia. It is extremely safe, and patients often feel great after surgery, just as if they have had a great night's sleep. Under local anesthesia, the awake nose job patient can swallow and clear the blood away with a handheld suction device during surgery. But because you are sleeping during twilight anesthesia, you cannot do this and your windpipe can become blocked with a blood clot. One way we modify a twilight type of anesthesia is in

> The value in not having general anesthesia is that it decreases the amount of bleeding during surgery and therefore bruising and postoperative recovery is lessened.

rhinoplasty cases. Here, we place a dam called an LMA (Laryngeal Mask Anesthesia) in the back of the throat to prevent blood from dripping into the windpipe. This is an important modification that I suggest any patient discuss with his or her surgeon prior to having a rhinoplasty surgery under twilight anesthesia.

Many plastic surgeons will perform surgery only under general anesthesia. I do agree that the risks of having serious complications after anesthesia are extremely low (less than .001 percent); however, there is no question that the rate of nausea, discomfort, and the increased bruising associated with general anesthesia warrant these surgeons reconsider their approach. In my opinion, the reason surgeons continue to do surgery exclusively under general anesthesia has more to do with the doctor's comfort in performing surgery with the patient asleep than what's the best option for the patient.

References

Tse, M.M., M.F. Chan, I.F. Benzie. 2005. The effect of music therapy on postoperative pain, heart rate, systolic blood pressures and analgesic use following nasal surgery. *Journal of Pain and Palliative Care Pharmacotherapy.* 19(3): 21-29.

10 Preparing for Surgery and Enhancing Healing

Faster healing time is among the top concerns of facial plastic surgery patients because they are usually very busy and are eager to return to their public lives as quickly as possible. Until recently, patients desiring a younger or aesthetically more balanced look have had to submit to a procedure such as a facelift that required a two- to three-week recovery and a risk of visible scarring. My coordinated approach to healing uses homeopathic medicines and even sometimes incorporates hyperbaric oxygen therapy so that patients can return to their lives looking refreshed and more youthful in five to seven days.

One way to minimize recovery time is to seek out a highly skilled facial plastic surgeon who employs minimal incision approaches and less-traumatic techniques which reduce recovery time. These techniques will be described in chapters that lie ahead.

As important as your choice of surgeon is how well you prepare for your surgery. All patients should have a complete physical examination by their internist (not their plastic surgeon) to assess their physical wellness and preparedness for surgery. A simple example is that poorly controlled high blood pressure can result in excessive bleeding after surgery and hence more bruising and swelling. Medications that are prescribed by your physician that will thin the blood or inhibit surgical healing should be substituted.

With this completed, I start my patients on a strict regimen *two weeks prior to surgery*. The first thing patients must do is avoid medications, supplements, and habits that reduce the body's ability to stop bleeding during surgery, which will inevitably increase post-procedure bruising, swelling, and recovery time.

Medications to Discontinue

- *Aspirin, Plavix, Coumadin,* and anti-inflammatories, such as over-the-counter drugs Advil, Motrin, Aleve, Naproxen, either impair platelet function or protein production necessary for clotting. Be aware that most cold remedies contain these drugs. Tylenol (acetaminophen) is the only safe painkiller in the preoperative period.

- *Vitamin E* can thin the blood and cause more bleeding and bruising. Many health foods, shakes, and energy bars have excessive vitamin E.

- *Omega-3s and fish oils* are nutritional supplements that inhibit clotting and can increase bleeding during surgery.

- *Ginkgo biloba* has an anticoagulant effect and causes bleeding.

- *Willow bark* is an herbal supplement that contains salicin, which is a precursor of aspirin.

Stop Smoking

Smoking increases swelling, limits blood flow to the skin during healing, and worsens scarring. If you smoke, you need to refrain from smoking two weeks before and two weeks after surgery. That means no nicotine for one month, including no nicotine gums to curb cravings because nicotine negatively affects healing. Due to the difficulty of the task, I often give patients a prescriptive medicine such as Chantix that helps them kick the habit short-term. There is a light at the end of the tunnel for smokers, as they can return to this destructive habit later if they choose. I am pleased that patients will often stop smoking permanently after surgery; the surgery was the catalyst to cessation. There is a dual benefit to stop smoking permanently: Not only are you healthier overall, but the results of the surgical procedure will last about twice as long in a nonsmoker.

Avoid Alcohol

Alcohol intake should be avoided completely for two weeks before surgery. Alcohol thins the blood and can increase bleeding during surgery. More bleeding increases the duration of bruising after surgery.

Other Presurgery Guidelines

There are other "housekeeping" items to address in the two weeks before surgery. Patients who color their hair should do so as close as possible to the date of surgery because their hair cannot be dyed again until four weeks after surgery. All medications should be purchased and available at home before surgery. All postoperative instruction sheets should be reviewed and available at home to refer to after surgery.

Your surgeon's instructions will also include this important notice: *Do not eat after midnight the day before surgery. If you do eat, your procedure must be delayed.* If your stomach has food in it, you may aspirate (vomit) while you are asleep.

Finally, wear a comfortable outfit to surgery, usually a sweat pants, with a shirt that zips or buttons down the front so that it will not be necessary to pull it over your face after your procedure.

Enhancing Post-Surgical Recovery

Homeopathy

Now that your body has been prepared for the surgery, there are three major ways—during and after the surgery—to enhance recovery. As mentioned, avoiding general anesthesia speeds healing because general anesthesia results in dilation of blood vessels leading to more bleeding during, and more bruising after, surgery, as described in chapter 9. After the surgery, homeopathic and nutritional supplements that have been proven in clinical studies to improve healing should be introduced. Hyperbaric oxygen therapy treatments can be incorporated postoperatively for their ability to speed healing. These treatments involve the patient breathing pure oxygen while he or she is in a sealed chamber that has been pressurized at 1½ to 3 times the normal atmospheric pressure.

Homeopathy is a system of natural health care that has been in worldwide use for more than 2,000 years. It is recognized by the World Health Organization as the second-largest therapeutic system in use in the world. While it is most popular in India and South America, more than 30 million people in Europe and millions of others around the world also benefit from its use.

Homeopathy is founded on the principle of "like cures like." The body knows what it is doing and symptoms are the body's way of taking action to overcome illness. This healing response is automatic in living organisms. Homeopathic medicine acts as a stimulus to the natural vital response, giving it the information it needs to complete its healing work.

Scientific studies indicate that homeopathic remedies like arnica montana and dietary supplements like bromelain and hyaluronic acid can help minimize swelling and bruising and speed healing. I have been prescribing homeopathic remedies to my own patients for years. What I have found to be most difficult is for my patients to find the exact supplements and homeopathic treatments at their local nutrition store and at the correct strength and formulation.

That is why I created the J Pak Systems. J Pak Systems is a homeopathic healing supplement system that provides an all-in-one, convenient solution featuring precise doses of the most refined, concentrated, bioavailable formulas in single-dose packets. J Pak No. 1 is for

> **Scientific studies indicate that homeopathic remedies like arnica montana and dietary supplements like bromelain and hyaluronic acid can help minimize swelling and bruising and speed healing.**

use before and after aesthetic injectable treatments to minimize bruising and swelling; J Pak No. 2 is for use after plastic surgery to optimize healing.

Both J Pak No. 1 and J Pak No. 2 contain arnica montana and bromelain. Arnica montana, or leopard's bane, a perennial herb indigenous to central Europe, has long been used to reduce posttraumatic bruising and swelling. In fact, published studies indicate that arnica montana can significantly reduce these effects. Bromelain is an enzyme derived from pineapple stems with anti-inflammatory properties. Published studies indicate that bromelain reduced edema (swelling) and ecchymosis (bruising) following surgical and nonsurgical trauma to the face.

J Pak No. 2 contains other nutritional supplements required for healing, including hyaluronic acid, glucosamine, vitamin C, and zinc.

The supplements regimen is started three days before surgery to get the body fueled for the healing process and then continued for two weeks after surgery. Hyaluronic acid is a carbohydrate component of the extracellular (outside the cells) matrix of skin and is secreted during wound and tissue repair. It is produced by fibroblasts (cells in the skin) during wound repair. Published studies indicate that hyaluronic

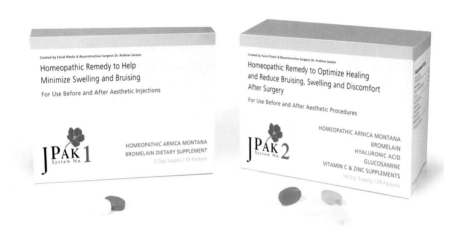

Figure 21. JPak Systems Homeopathic Healing Supplement Systems are used to reduce bruising from facial injections and from cosmetic surgery.

acid helps accelerate healing. Glucosamine compounds have been reported to have several beneficial effects on the skin and its cells. Because it stimulates hyaluronic acid synthesis, it has also been shown to accelerate wound healing, improve skin hydration, and decrease wrinkles. Vitamin C is an essential cofactor for collagen production and wound healing which requires the production of new collagen. Zinc is an essential trace element in the human body. It serves as a cofactor in skin cell migration during wound repair.

Whether you are having noninvasive or more-invasive treatments to enhance your facial appearance, the J Pak Systems can help speed your recovery and enjoy your results earlier. J Pak System products can be purchased at www.jpaksystems.com.

Hyperbaric Oxygen Therapy

Until now, homeopathy was the only way to increase the speed of healing and get back to your work and social life more quickly. I performed a study to identify whether hyperbaric oxygen (HBO) therapy would increase how quickly my patients heal. HBO works to increase oxygen to facial tissue and stimulate the growth of new blood vessels, which in turn contributes to a faster recovery. In this study, patients underwent HBO therapy for two days before their facelift surgery and three days after surgery. The study showed that hyperbaric oxygen decreases bruising by 35 percent at one week after surgery.

Hyperbaric oxygen therapy offers patients an additional option for quicker recovery from facelift surgery and potentially other cosmetic procedures. It is an excellent tool for patients with limited available recovery time for faster resolution of postoperative swelling and bruising. It works to increase oxygen to facial tissue and stimulate the growth of new blood vessels, which, in turn, contributes to a faster recovery.

References

Desneves, K.J., B.E. Todorovic, A. Cassar, T.C. Crowe. 2005. Treatment with supplementary arginine, vitamin C and zinc in patients with pressure ulcers: A randomized controlled trial. *Clinical Nutrition.* Dec; 24(6): 979-987.

Kamenicek, V. et al. 2001. Systemic enzyme therapy in the treatment and prevention of post-traumatic and postoperative swelling. *Acta Chirurgiae Orthopaedicae et Traumatologiae Cechoslovaca.* 68(1): 45-49.

McCarty, M.F. 1996. Glucosamine for wound healing. *Medical Hypotheses.* Oct;47(4): 273-275

Parikh, S.S., A.A. Jacono. 2011. Deep-plane facelift as an alternative in the smoking patient. *Archives of Facial Plastic Surgery.* Jul-Aug; 13(4): 283-285.

Seeley, B.M., A.B. Denton, M.S. Ahn, C.S. Maas. 2006. Effect of homeopathic arnica montana on bruising in facelifts: results of a randomized, double-blind, placebo-controlled clinical trial. Archives of Facial Plastic Surgery. Jan-Feb; 8(1):54-59.

Seltzer, A.P. 1964. A double-blinded study of Bromelain in the treatment of edema and ecchymosis following surgical and nonsurgical trauma to the face. *Eye Ear Nose Throat Monthly.* 43: 54.

Totonchi, A., B. Guyuron. 2007. A randomized, controlled comparison between arnica and steroids in the management of postrhinoplasty ecchymosis and edema. *Plastic Reconstuctive Surgery.* Jul; 120(1): 271-274.

Voinchet, V., P. Vasseur, and J. Kern. Efficacy and safety of hyaluronic acid in the management of acute wounds. *American Journal of Clinical Dermatology.* 206; 7(6) 353-357.

11 Younger-Looking Eyes and Brows

It is said that the eyes are the windows to the soul. Your eyelid and brow appearance are the first things people notice when they meet you, because when we communicate, we look into each other's eyes. Droopy upper eyelids are the results of excess sagging eyelid skin and can make you look tired, angry, or just older. People will often describe "hooding" of their upper eyelids and difficulty applying eyelid makeup to the upper eyelid crease. The skin gets in the way and also washes the makeup off over a short period of time during normal blinking. Sometime the hooding is so severe that it can block vision.

This can happen at a very early age, as there are familial patterns of aging; I have performed upper eyelid surgery in women as young as thirty years old. Younger patients often tell me that they started noticing the changes in their twenties and that everyone in their family has the same upper eyelid appearance.

Sometimes the upper eyelids appear droopy, but the problem is not with the upper eyelids but with the forehead and brow. When the forehead drops, the eyebrows fall in front of the upper eyelids like a window shade. You can do as much work as you like on the window (eyelids) but if the window shade (eyebrows and brow skin) is blocking the window, you will never see the window. The best way to decide for yourself is to sit in front of the mirror and lift your forehead just above the eyebrows, giving them a lift. If you like what you see, you do not need an upper eyelid lift, but a brow lift. In some people, both an upper eyelid lift and a brow lift should be executed at the same time to give the best result, but this can best be determined by your plastic surgeon.

With age, the lower eyelids become puffy and bags develop due to prolapse of fat underneath the eyes. At the same time, dark circles and hollowness, called "tear troughs," develop under these bags. This is the result of volume loss along the cheekbones and the drooping of the cheeks, creating under-eye circles. There are many different surgical and nonsurgical approaches to improve these conditions, but in this chapter I will focus on the surgical solutions. Nonsurgical eyelid lift approaches are discussed in chapter 5.

The surgeon should evaluate the eyelids and brow through the eyes of both a surgeon and an artist. Beautiful, youthful eyes have a relationship (the Golden Proportion of beauty is discussed in chapter 2) between the eyebrows and eyelids. The ratio of the distance from the eyebrow at its highest outer arch to the upper eyelashes is ideally 1.618 times (Φ) the distance from the lower eyelid lashes to the beginning of the cheek; this is a Golden Proportion. As we age our eyelid proportions change.

Older brows droop over the eyes, causing the upper eyelids to shorten, throwing off the Golden Proportion of youth. When lower eyelids hollow and cheeks droop, dark circles under the eyes are created, and the lower eyelid lengthens. In fact, the combination of lowering of the upper eyelid and lengthening of the lower eyelid actually creates the inverse or opposite of the Golden Ratio of youth and beauty.

Restoring the Upper Eyelid Crease

If your brow and lower eyelid proportions are good, then all that would be necessary is an upper eyelid lift, or as doctors call it, an upper blepharoplasty.

In upper eyelid lift surgery, incisions are placed in the natural eyelid crease to keep the incisions as invisible as possible along these natural folds. The location of these incisions is marked with the patient sitting upright and the eyes closed. This allows for precise location of the incisions and calculation of the amount of extra skin to be removed that still allows the upper eyelids to close.

If a doctor marks a patient in a position lying down, then he or she might take away too much skin and the patient would not be able to close their eyes. This creates a condition of severe dry eyes. The incisions must go past the outer corner of the eye and continue into a natural crow's foot wrinkle so that all the hooded skin under the eyebrow can be removed. If the incision stops short at the outer corner

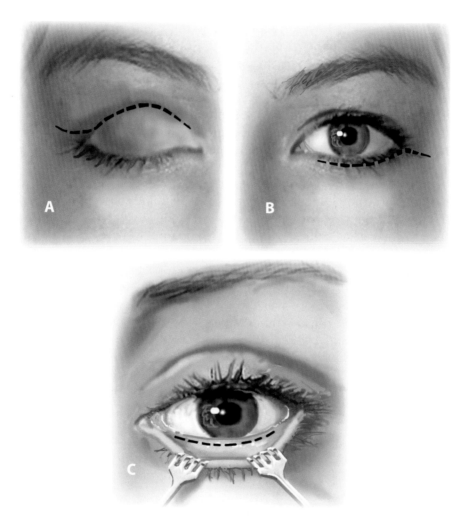

Figures 22A, 22B, 22C. Location of eyelid lift incisions. A) The incision for an upper eyelid lift is hidden in the upper eyelid crease and a "crow's foot" wrinkle. B) Incision for a lower eyelid lift to remove excess skin is placed two mm below the eyelashes. C) Lower eyelid incision from inside the eyelid, called a "trans-conjunctival" incision, is used when fat bags under the eyes need work but no skin removal is necessary.

of the eye, bunching of the extra hooded skin that is left behind looks like "curtain call" drapery at the end of a Broadway show. This is not a good look!

After excision of the skin, the extra fat pads of the upper eyelid are removed, but we want to remove only what is excessive and not remove all the fat. The most common bulge of fat requiring removal in the upper eyelid is at the inner corner by the nose. If all the fat pad in the center of the upper eyelid is removed, the upper eyelid appears longer than normal. This would make the ratio of the upper eyelid length to the lower eyelid length larger than the Golden Proportion, and make the upper eyelids look altered and plastic.

Endoscopic or Keyhole Brow Techniques

When upper eyelids are heavy, and it has been determined that it is a result of the forehead drooping over the upper eyelids, a brow-lift surgery is indicated.

As we previously discussed, beautiful and natural eyebrow position respects the Golden Proportion. The eyebrow starts at the level of the inner corner of the eye. At this point the vertical height of the eyebrow should be where the forehead bone starts. The length of the eyebrow from left to right should be 1.618 times the Golden Ratio the distance between the inner corners of the left and right eyes (this is called the intercanthal distance). There should be a gentle upward curve to the brow's lateral tip that should be placed .618 of the intercanthal distance above the bone underneath the eyebrow. Patients are scared of brow-lift surgery because they often see people looking unnaturally startled or surprised after this procedure. This is especially true when the eyebrow position near the nose is higher or at the same height as its outer tip. In this case, the Golden Proportion of the eyebrow is not respected because there should be an outer tilt to the eyebrow. This commonly occurs from a traditional brow lift that most doctors still execute (but I do not). Further, this looks odd because the overly elevated brow makes the upper eyelid appears longer than normal. These two problems are why Kenny Rogers looks so altered after presumed plastic surgery.

In the traditional brow lift, an incision is used that runs across the top of the head, from one ear to the other. This is a long incision, and the invasive nature of this procedure results in prominent scarring and a longer recovery. Side effects include numbness of the scalp that feels like there is a permanent cap on the top of the head.

An endoscopic or keyhole brow lift is the more appropriate way to accomplish the goals of forehead lifting surgery, which is to create balance. Endoscopic simply means "telescopic." Through a few small incisions in the hairline just large enough to pass the endoscope (which is the width of a drinking straw), the surgery is accomplished. It is the same concept as telescopic gallbladder excisions: years ago when doctors removed your gallbladder, they made an incision that was a

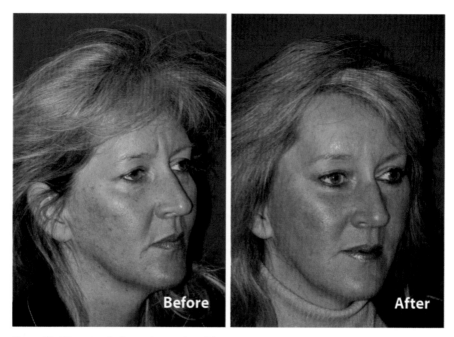

Figure 23. This patient had an endoscopic browlift. During surgery, the muscle between the eyes is relaxed to remove frown lines. The eyebrows are elevated subtlety to open the eyes. The "keyhole" incisions are hidden in the hairline.

foot long under the rib cage. Now, with a few small incisions and a telescope, the same surgery is performed with a quicker recovery and less scarring.

With the keyhole technique, the forehead, including the skin and muscle, is lifted off the bone. The layer that attaches the overlying tissues to the bone is the periosteum. This burlap-like layer, like a supporting cable, is the one that weakens as you get older and allows the tissues to drop. The eyebrows are detached from the orbital (eye socket) bone, so they can be gently lifted, and the corrugator supercilli muscle that causes the frown lines between the eyebrows is released.

The frown lines are then permanently reversed, obviating the need for future botulinum toxin injections here. The tissues are then lifted and held into their elevated position with sutures. In this surgery, we never lift the center of the brows much, if at all, because this is what creates the startled appearance of older brow lifts. The outer edge of the eyebrow, also called the tail of the brow, is elevated, which creates a natural and feminine appearance and respects a Golden Relationship between the upper and lower eyelids.

I do not suggest brow-lifting surgery in the vast majority of men as they age. When we look at the brow position of iconic leading men in Hollywood who are considered to be very attractive, like Brad Pitt and Tom Cruise, we notice that they have heavy brows. A heavier brow accentuates the bridge of bone in the forehead right above the eyes that doctors call the supraorbital ridge. This is a male facial skeletal characteristic. Since this is accentuated with age, it is one of the reasons that men are seen to be more handsome and distinguished as they get older. Additionally, brows orientation in men should go straight across this part of the forehead, as it also accentuates this bony ridge. The brows should not arch up above the bone because this is a female orientation for the brows.

To perform a brow lift on men would reduce the masculinity of the face. In fact, raising the brows would feminize the face. Brow lifting is why many male celebrities look so odd after plastic surgery. In men, I usually perform only upper eyelid surgery for heavier, tired upper eyes, and reserve brow lifts for those cases where the brows have fallen low enough that they start to obstruct vision.

An endoscopic or keyhole brow lift offers the advantage of a quick recovery phase. The recovery time is usually five to seven days. All incisions are hidden behind the hairline so that they are not visible to anyone.

Lower Eyelid Lift—Where Fat Transposition Fits In

There are two ways to perform a lower eyelid lift, one that requires an external incision in the skin and the other that requires an internal incision inside the eye. The approach that is chosen is dependent upon whether excess skin needs to be removed or if just the fat bags under the eyes need to be treated. The external incision technique is used when extra skin needs to be removed, and the incision is placed just underneath (two millimeters below) the lower eyelash line. This gives access to the lower eyelid excessive muscle and fat and allows the skin to be trimmed and tightened. Extremely fine sutures are then used to meticulously close the incisions, thus minimizing the visibility of any scar. The "scarless" technique, called a transconjunctival blepharoplasty, places an incision inside the eyelid through the lining of the eye (the conjunctiva) to access the redundant muscle and fat. This technique is used on younger patients who have not yet developed excess skin. Sometimes a chemical peel or laser resurfacing, as described in chapter 7, will tighten the surface of the skin when combined with a scarless lower eyelid lift.

In the vast majority of lower eyelid surgery cases, it is important not to remove the fat bags under the eyes, but rather transpose or move the fat into the deep grooving and hollows that appear as dark circles. When fat bags are removed from the lower eyelids, it creates a hollowing effect that is a telltale sign of surgery.

As part of the natural aging process, the area underneath the lower eyelid bags hollows, and the cheeks droop, making the lower eyelid appear to lengthen. Removing fat makes the lower eyelid's perceived length increase and look older, but in a different way. Because part of getting older is losing the natural volume of the face, refilling the deflated eyelid and cheek junction defines a more youthful appearance. Since the fat is left attached to the blood supply around the eye, these fat pads, which are stitched into position and cannot move, will last a lifetime. This is different from fat transfers that are removed from the belly or thighs and injected into these hollows. In my experience, these transfers reabsorb and go away 33 percent of the time.

Revision Eyelid Surgery

Sometimes, initial surgery of the eyes does not deliver the desired result, requiring revision procedures. Unsatisfactory results following blepharoplasty or eyelid lift surgery require very specialized surgical techniques. The delicate tissues of the eyelid are notoriously unforgiving in their response to overzealous surgery; consequently, revision blepharoplasty must be precise and delicate. While many flaws may resolve with time (three to six months or more), more resistant difficulties may sometimes require further revision blepharoplasty surgery. There are two different types of revision eyelid surgery. One is to perform revision blepharoplasty for undercorrection where extra eyelid skin and bags are left behind, and the other is to perform revision eyelid lift surgery when too much skin and fat was removed, creating an unnatural look where the eyes look sunken and change shape.

Revision surgery can correct an uneven appearance of the eyes. In upper and lower eyelid surgery this usually means removing excess skin and fat that were left behind. In the upper eyelid, the most common place to leave extra fat is in area by the junction of the corner of upper eyelid and the nose, and the most common place to leave extra skin is in the hooding of the outer corner of the upper eyelid. In the lower eyelid surgery the most common place to leave extra bulges behind is in the outer corner; they look like a pea or cyst.

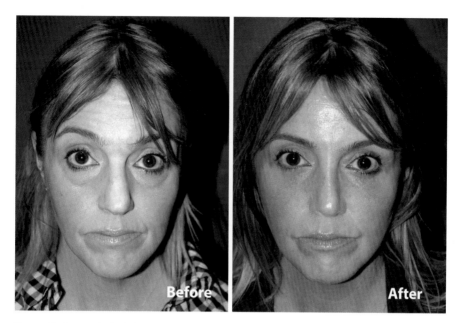

Figure 24. Patient who had a lower eyelid lift with transposition (moving) of the fat bags into the lower eyelid circles. She also had rhinoplasty at the same time.

Severe tissue shortage or scarring from prior surgery may require extensive reconstructive surgery. In an upper eyelid lift, sometimes too much skin is removed and the patient cannot close his or her eyes. In this case, a doctor must perform skin grafts to the upper eyelids. Other times, if upper blepharoplasty is overdone, the muscle that opens the eye, the levator muscle, can be damaged or partially removed by being too aggressive. This is called ptosis and an operation called a ptosis repair is performed, during which the muscle is reconstructed and tightened.

The most common problem in lower blepharoplasty, however, is ectropion, where the eyelid gets pulled down, and the shape of the eye becomes rounded and less almond-shaped. I have pioneered surgical techniques to deal with this problem. Ectropion repair techniques include lateral canthal surgery, which changes the lower eyelid tendons, as well as endoscopic mid-face surgery, which helps support the lower eyelids by lifting the cheeks. If too much fat is removed from the eyes, a fat transfer or fat grafting from the abdomen to the under-eye region is often necessary.

References

Baker, S.R. 1999. Orbital fat preservation in lower-lid blepharo-plasty. *Archives of Facial Plastic Surgery.* 1(1): 33-37.

Jacono, A.A., B. Stong. 2010. Combined transconjunctival release and mid-facelift for postblepharoplasty ectropion repair. *Archives of Facial Plastic Surgery.* May-Jun; 12(3): 206-208.

Jacono, A.A., B. Moskowitz. 2001. Transconjunctival versus transcutaneous approach in upper and lower blepharoplasty. *Facial Plastic Surgery.* Feb; 17(1): 21-28.

Marten, T.J. 2008. Closed, nonendoscopic, small-incision fore-head lift. *Clinical Plastic Surgery.* Jul; 35(3): 363-378.

Romo, III, T., A.A. Jacono, A.P. Sclafani. 2001. Endoscopic fore-head lifting and contouring. *Facial Plastic Surgery.* Feb; 17(1): 3-10.

12 Facial Rejuvenation: Lifting the Face and Neck

Long-standing facelifting techniques with larger incisions do not restore the youthful volume in the arc of the eyes and the cheeks. The result is a sculpted, stretched look and scarring—the telltale signs of plastic surgery. My new facelift approach focuses on rebuilding and lifting the foundation of the face, not stretching the surface, thus avoiding these problems.

Do You Hate Your Neck?

At some point nearly every woman, and also every man, will tug on the slack skin under his or her neck and wish it were gone. The most common ages to request surgery for loosening of the face ranges from the late forties to the seventies. The main factors that I see bring patients to consider a facelifting surgery are whether they are aging prematurely and looking older than their years (for example looking fifty-five years old and actually being forty-five) or because their tolerance for aging differs (for example a woman who has had a heavy neck since the age of sixty but waits until she is seventy-eight to have her first facelift).

As I stated in chapter 6, although there is no exact age when the face needs to be supported by a lifting procedure, the most common age women seek a consultation is fifty-four years old, which is on average three years after they experience menopause. After three years without estrogen stimulation of the face, the quality of the skin changes significantly and the facial muscles loosen more in three years than in the prior fifty. In older faces, it is not enough to simply fill the face (for example with temporary fillers or fat transfers) because when the facial tissues have become too loose they cannot support the additional volume.

The goal of aging-face surgery is to reestablish the heart-shaped face of youth. In chapter 2, I described how a beautiful youthful face has a width between the cheekbones that is wider than the horizontal distance of the jaw—the Golden Proportion (1.618 to 1). As we age, jowls form on either side of the chin, making this horizontal length of the lower face wider, and "marionette lines," or grooves between the corner of the mouth and chin, develop.

This is accompanied by a "double chin" or "turkey gobbler" and vertical folds or bands in the neck. The cheeks deflate and the horizontal distance between them becomes shorter. These drooped cheeks create folding between the nose and mouth called nasolabial folds. To restore the natural beauty of youth and reestablish the Golden Proportion, a combination of lifting the jowls to reduce the width of the face along the jawline and repositioning the cheek higher to add width along the cheekbones is necessary.

There are corporate-sponsored facelifts that are advertised on television claiming no downtime, trademarked lifts (ones created with interesting names for advertising and marketing purposes), mini-lifts, S-lifts, MACS lifts, SMAS lifts, and deep plane lifts. This is all very confusing, and most people do not understand the inherent differences of these techniques. How do you decide what procedure gives the best results, with minimal scarring and downtime, and the longest lasting results? This is the most commonly asked question by my patients. I perform all types of facelifts for patients as it is not a one-size-fits-all approach, but it is important for patients to understand the pros and cons of different approaches so they can make an educated decision.

Short Scar, S-Lift, and Mini-Facelifts

A mini-facelift is a popular method to rejuvenate the lower third of the face, and it is also called a short scar facelift or an S-Lift. It is called an S-lift because the shape of the smaller incision used is that of an S. It starts hidden in the sideburn hair, runs just inside the ear canal, and ends just behind the earlobe without running into the scalp skin behind the ear. This is different from a traditional facelift scar that is usually twice as long, runs up higher into the scalp above the ear, and runs onto the scalp skin behind the ear. The S-lift incision is relatively well hidden; it is often called a "ponytail lift" because you can put your hair up in a ponytail without having visible scars behind the ears, as with a traditional facelift.

In a mini-lift, the skin is then elevated like in a traditional facelift. The muscle layer underneath the skin in the face and neck are the

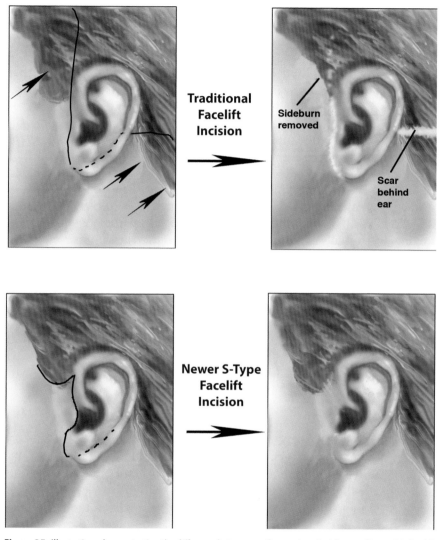

Figure 25. Illustrations demonstrating the difference between an S-type short incision used in a mini-facelift and the traditional facelift incision that is twice as long and not as well hidden.

SMAS and the platysma, respectively. These supportive muscles are not elevated off the face, but are simply tightened with stitches. This is called plication or imbrication sutures in doctor language. The jowls are corrected, but improvement in the neck is usually not complete. This greater improvement in the face compared to the neck looks like the wrong lid on a jar.

Because the muscles, which are the foundation of the face, are not lifted and re-supported but simply stitched, the majority of the tightening is on the skin surface that was elevated. The result can leave patients with a windswept, stretched, or pulled appearance. This is often why patients who have had a facelift *look* like they have had a facelift, often seen as pulling of the corners of the mouth. There is a lack of strength in the repair of a mini-lift as it relies mostly on the relatively thin skin, and results last only three to five years. The facial muscles are the structure of the face, the beams that hold up the facelift if you will, and if only lifted by placing some stitches on their surface, the face will fall earlier than desired.

What compounds this problem is that most facelifts of all types usually tighten the face along the jawline in a mostly horizontal direction. This is unnatural because the face falls vertically with gravity. Pulling horizontally across the face will flatten the cheeks, worsening the deflated-appearing cheeks of an older face. Although it can improve the jowls, the nasolabial folds remain unchanged. In order to improve the cheek appearance, fat transfers are often done, as described in chapter 6. This can be an effective technique if performed well, but fat transfers have the downside of the fat reabsorbing 33 percent of the time.

When the excess skin is removed from the horizontal dimension, the sideburns are often cut away, which is a telltale sign of a facelift. This becomes difficult to hide and requires creative camouflaging with hairstyling, especially as you cannot wear your hair back.

SMAS Facelifts

The difference between the mini-facelifts and SMAS facelifts is the incision and amount of work done to the underlying muscle of the face. SMAS lifts usually have a longer incision that continues onto the scalp skin behind the ear in order to perform more work on the neck. After the skin is lifted, the SMAS muscles, which exist in the lower face along the jowl region, and platysma muscle in the neck, are not simply stitched but are lifted, giving the face more support. SMAS techniques do not release the muscles of the cheeks because these muscles are different from the SMAS and are not part of the SMAS operation. The neck results are better, and the lifts have been shown to last around ten to twelve years. They still suffer from lack of improvement in the cheeks because they are a horizontally oriented tightening procedure and the cheek muscles are not released. Because the skin is separated from the muscle it still has a tendency to appear more tight or "plastic" on the surface.

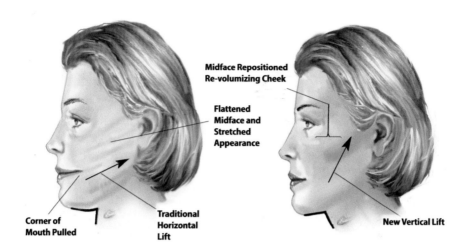

Figure 26. Illustration demonstrating how traditional facelifting (left) tightens the face horizontally, flattening the face and cheeks leaving a "lifted" appearance, versus a vertical oriented lift (right) that supports the cheeks, repositioning them upward. The vertical lift recreates the "apple cheeks" of youth.

Deep Plane Facelifts

A deep plane facelift is similar to the SMAS facelift with respect to the incision and the more horizontally directed tightening, but it differs in that the skin is never separated from the underlying muscle layer; the skin and muscle are lifted as one unit. Because the skin is never separated in a deep plane lift, these patients get less bruising. The SMAS and mini-lifts described above separate the skin more superficially and the bleeding and bruising are more visible as you recover.

Another difference in the deep plane lift is that the cheek muscles are released as part of this technique. Because the surgery places the tightening on the deeper muscle layer that is not separated from the skin, the face appears more natural and unstretched. Like a SMAS lift, these lifts usually last ten to twelve years. Even though the cheek muscles are released, this is still a more horizontal-based lift, and there are some mild but not dramatic changes in the cheek.

Interestingly, deep plane lifts are the only facelift type that can be performed safely on smokers. I have performed studies showing this to be a fact. This is because the skin and muscle are not separated, so the blood supply to the lifted tissues is better. The nicotine in cigarettes narrows the blood vessels in the skin. If the skin is separated as described in SMAS and mini-lifts, the skin can necrose or die off, which results in weeks of healing and bad scars.

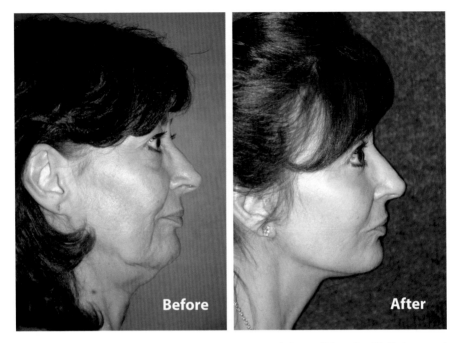

Figure 27. Patient who had a Minimal Access Deep Plane Extended Vertical Vector Facelift. Notice natural tightening along the neck and jawline as well as gentle lifting of the cheeks. Below, the close up view of the ear shows the S-type incision is not visible.

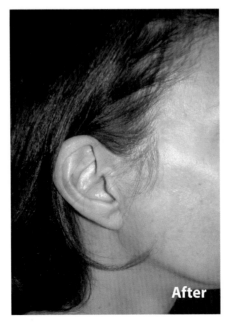

The MADE Lift:
Minimal Access Deep Plane Extended Facelift

The most state-of-the-art facelift is a hybrid technique that I developed called the MADE lift. It is a vertically oriented lift that works against the normal gravitational changes of aging. Additionally, it fuses the optimal features of older-generation, short-incision "mini" facelifts with the benefits of the muscle support of deep plane facelifts. Because it is a vertically oriented tightening, it supports the drooped cheeks, restoring volume to the cheekbones and smoothing nasolabial folds. This results in a youthful, beautiful, heart-shaped face that respects the Golden Proportion. Vertical vector lifting was first described in mini facelifts by Belgian plastic surgeons Patrick Tonnard and Alex Verpaele that only tightened the muscles with stitches; this is called a MACS lift.

The MADE lift uses a short S-type incision as described above, while lifting the facial tissue and muscles as one unit, so patients get the superior results of a deep plane facelift combined with the minimal scarring of a mini-lift. It is not only an option that delivers best-in-class results, but it is offers longer-lasting results as well. The standard lifetime of a mini-lift is between three to five years, but because the MADE lift relies on the support of a deep plane facelift, results last ten to twelve years. For years, my patients have had to choose between better results or less scarring. With this hybrid facelift, they get the best of both worlds. In patients with advanced aging and heavier necks, a hybrid lift can still be performed, but the incision length is increased.

Given the level of difficulty in performing this procedure, because a more detailed understanding of the anatomy is required, I encourage any patient considering this procedure to seek a physician who specializes in facial plastic surgery and possesses the level of expertise required to perform a hybrid facelift. I review how to select the best surgeon in chapter 17.

The Endoscopic Mid-Facelift

For those patients who do not require any improvement of the jawline and neck, there is a minimally invasive surgical procedure to lift the drooped cheeks called an endoscopic mid-facelift. This is most commonly performed on women and men in their forties to early fifties.

Endoscopic mid-facelifting utilizes only two small incisions hidden in the hairline just big enough to insert an endoscope the size of a drinking straw. The cheeks' deep tissues including the muscles and cheek fat pad called the malar fat pad are lifted off the cheekbones

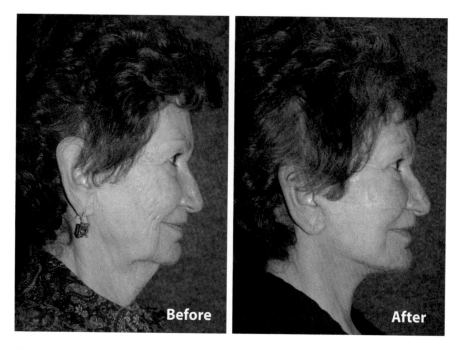

Figure 28. Patient with advanced aging and a heavy neck who had a MADE facelift.

and repositioned. This less-invasive facelift technique, combined with reestablishing the fat pads, restores the heart-shaped face of youth. An endoscopic mid-facelift has the advantage of having a shorter recovery (five to seven days) than the facelifts described above (ten to fourteen days), and lasts usually five to ten years.

Minor Neck Procedures

For those with less neck drooping, a smaller, isolated neck surgery can be performed. There are three components that make the neck look heavy: extra fat under the chin, vertical banding of the platysma in the neck, and loose skin.

Excess fat deposits beneath the chin can occur in women and men of all ages, creating an undesirable contour or making the neck appear to hang. This area can be sculpted to produce a smoother, more attractive neck and jawline by using liposuction. To remove the fat, a tiny incision is made beneath the chin and behind each ear. Using a small device called a cannula, the fat is suctioned away. As the fat is removed, it separates the skin from the underlying muscle. As the skin heals, it contracts and tightens up. This works only with patients

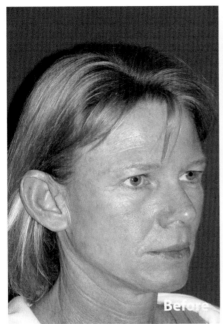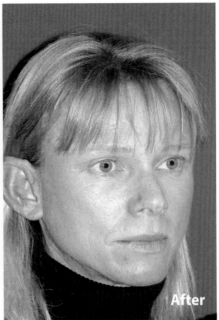

Figure 29. Patient who had an endoscopic midface lift to re-create the heart-shaped face of youth by lifting the cheeks. She also had an upper and lower eyelid lift at the same time.

without a lot of extra skin, or else it is like deflating a balloon and the skin will hang more.

If there is loosening of the platysma muscle in the neck, a small incision is made under the chin, extra fat that contributes to the "turkey gobbler" is removed and the platysma muscle (the muscle that separates in the center, causing vertical bands in the neck) is tightened with sutures. This is called a platysmoplasty, and, as in liposuction, is best performed when only smaller amounts of extra skin exist under the chin.

If there is a lot of extra skin under the neck, an isolated neck lift can be performed through an incision behind the ears only. The platysma muscle is also tightened during this surgery and the extra skin is cut away.

Revision Facelift Surgery

Revision facelifts or secondary facelifts are procedures done after a person has already had a facelift. My practice specializes in revision facelift surgery and corrective facelift surgery. Generally, patients who

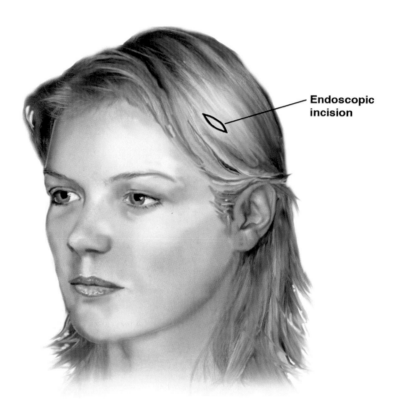

Endoscopic
incision

Figure 30. Illustration showing the incision placement for an endoscopic mid-facelift to lift the cheeks and central portions of the face. There is no visible scarring—the incision is hidden inside the hairline.

consult me for revision facelift procedures have significantly different needs from the patients who have not had prior facial rejuvenation surgery. As a result, a revision or corrective facelift requires special techniques and care because of previous surgical manipulations. In these cases, I use a customized approach that deals with the issues unique to each patient.

People seek revision facelifts for many reasons. The most common scenario: the person has had a successful facelift that has naturally aged over time, and now it is time to repeat it to maintain a youthful appearance. Most times, well-performed facelifts last more than ten years. Other times, a person has had a facelift and the result was not acceptable because areas of the face were undertreated. The most common problems include continued jowls or neck laxity after surgery, or drooping of the cheeks and mid-facial area after a facelift. Procedures that do not last as long as anticipated are also a very common reason a person will inquire about a secondary facelift procedure. Patients who were "overdone" and have a tight or stretched appearance tend to be dissatisfied and also seek corrective facelift revision procedures.

Any facelift technique that places excessive tightness on the skin can produce scarring and distortions, including pulling down of the earlobes (pixie ear deformity) or hairline problems (loss of sideburns). Although earlobe distortions can be fixed during a revision facelift, the only way to replace lost sideburns is with follicular unit hair transplantation, discussed in chapter 8.

Many patients who have undergone previous lifting procedures have thinner skin and require special treatment to avoid complications from secondary procedures. After the skin has been thoroughly evaluated, the facial balance between the upper, middle, lower, and neck regions of the face must all be detailed. The areas of imbalance can be addressed at the same time with an endoscopic brow lift, mid-facelift, or blepharoplasty procedures. Also, we now know that the aging process is not just a matter of gravitational laxity but that significant volume atrophy is present due to the change to the skeletal bone as well as subcutaneous fat atrophy. As a result, many patients undertaking secondary facial procedures will require multilevel fat transfer and grafting to restore facial volume, as discussed in chapter 6.

Facelift revision procedures must concentrate on the sagging deep tissue that has not been addressed by the original superficial facelift. In these cases, a deep plane facelift is indicated because it does not tighten the skin and is directed at the sagging deep tissue. It lifts under the SMAS and platysma muscle, supports the face, lifts drooping, and takes the tightness off the skin. It is the best option for a second facelift without producing any further tightening of the skin layer, and it will correct residual jowling, heavy neck, cheek drooping, and nasolabial folds in one procedure.

If the only problem is drooping cheeks, and the jawline and neck were corrected by the first facelift, an endoscopic mid-facelift is indicated. The endoscopic mid-facelift was developed by combining modern endoscopic techniques and craniofacial reconstruction and is utilized by only a few select surgeons around the world in facial cosmetic surgery. Using small incisions and a small telescope, the mid-face region is elevated and placed back in its original position. The eyelid-cheek regions, as well as the nasolabial folds, return to their natural youthful position, providing significant harmony to the face. The drooping cheeks, hollowness under the eyes, and smile or "laugh lines" can be dramatically improved.

Some people will complain about their scars but be satisfied with their facelift. Bad scars are always the result of excessive skin tightness. Simply cutting and re-suturing the scars alone (scar revision) will produce greater tension on the new scar and cause a worse resultant scar and should be avoided. In these situations, revising the facelift with a lift that supports the muscles and the deep layer of the face will allow the old scars to be removed and take the tension off the skin so the new incision lines will heal without bad scars. This is how we fix earlobes that are pulled down. This procedure actually requires revising the entire facelift and is not directed solely at the earlobe.

References

Baker, D.C. 2008. Lateral SMASectomy, plication and short scar facelifts: Indications and techniques. *Clinical Plastic Surgery*. 35: 533-550, vi.

Hamra, S.T. 1990. The deep-plane rhytidectomy. *Plastic and Reconstructive Surgery*. 86: 53-61; discussion 62-63.

Jacono, A.A., S.S. Parikh. 2011. The minimal access deep plane extended vertical facelift. *Aesthetic Surgery Journal*. Nov; 31(8): 874-890.

Parikh, S.S., A.A. Jacono. 2011. Deep plane facelift as an alternative in the smoking patient. *Archives of Facial Plastic Surgery*. Jul-Aug; 13(4): 283-285.

Prado, A., P. Andrades, S. Danilla, P. Castillo, P. Leniz. 2006. A clinical retrospective study comparing two short-scar facelifts: Minimal access cranial suspension versus lateral SMASectomy. *Plastic and Reconstructive Surgery*. 117: 1413-1425.

Quatela, V.C., A.A. Jacono. 2003. The extended centrolateral endoscopic mid-facelift. *Facial Plastic Surgery*. May; 19(2): 199-208.

Tonnard, P., A. Verpaele, S. Monstrey, et al. 2002. Minimal access cranial suspension lift: A modified S-lift. *Plastic and Reconstructive Surgery*. 109: 2074-2086.

13 Facial Recontouring: Cheeks and Chin

One of the strongest characteristics of youth is fullness of the cheeks, indicating an abundance of healthy soft tissues and healthy fat under the skin. Flat cheekbones can make a large nose look larger and a receding chin appear smaller. The cheekbones are largely responsible for defining your face, highlighting your eyes, and adding balance to your features. Altering your face's bony features improves your overall facial harmony and beauty dramatically.

Beautiful cheeks are defined by their height and volume; we often hear how people desire high cheekbones and appreciate youthful "apple cheeks" that have an oval volume. The ideal location of the cheek can be located by drawing a triangle around the three major landmarks that surround the cheek, as described in chapter 2 (see figure 8). The points of the triangle are from the corner of the mouth to the outer corner of the eye to the center of the ear.

The ideal location for a beautiful cheekbone lies along a line drawn from the corner of the eye to the base of this triangle in the Golden Proportion of 1.618 to 1. Creating the Golden Ratio in the cheeks will make the face more attractive by drawing attention to the eyes and cheeks, rather than to the lower face.

With age, you may lose fullness in your face, especially in the cheek area. If this has happened to you, you could be an ideal candidate for cheek augmentation. I believe that lifting this area with new, natural facelift and mid-facelift techniques, as discussed in chapter 12, or replacing the lost volume of the face with fat transfers, as discussed in chapter 6, creates a more natural appearance in older patients than an implant. Placing implants in a patient who has always had beautiful high cheekbones in youth can sometimes overly widen the upper face, creating a very masculine appearance. This represents a nonharmonious state as the ratio of the upper cheeks to the lower face would be greater than the Golden Ratio.

In 2011, nearly 8,000 cheek implant procedures were performed, according to statistics compiled by the American Society of Plastic Surgeons. There are two different ways to augment the cheeks: nonsurgically and surgically. Cheeks can be augmented nonsurgically with temporary fillers such as hyaluronic acids (Perlane, Juvederm, Restylane), Radiesse, and Sculptra Aesthetic. Fat transfer injects fat suctioned from the abdomen or thighs into the cheeks and is a minimally invasive procedure as it does not require incisions on the face and has a rapid recovery. How these procedures are performed is reviewed in chapters 4 and 5.

Cheek Augmentation

Surgical cheek augmentation is done using cheek implants (known to physicians as malar and submalar augmentation). The surgical use of sterile synthetics or biological implants is performed to bring the cheeks into better balance with other facial features. It is very common to have cheek implants when a nose job (rhinoplasty) is being done. The outcome should be a balanced relationship between the structures of the face.

With the increasing popularity of cosmetic surgery procedures, including cheek implants, it is important for prospective patients to research and understand different issues, such as what the procedure can and cannot offer, inherited risks, costs, and other factors. Keep in mind that cosmetic surgery is just that—a surgical procedure with results that cannot simply be erased. Sometimes, cheek implants are designed for facial reconstruction rather than rejuvenation. Regardless of the reason, you should understand the basic steps of a cheek implant procedure:

- To place cheek implants, a small incision is made near where the implant will be placed. The incision is made inside the mouth where your upper lip meets your gums.

- A pocket is then created over the actual cheekbone where the implant will be positioned. As always, this is not a one-size-fits all procedure. I often will place many different implant shapes and sizes into the pocket during surgery with "sizers" or test implants to ensure the implant is customized to the patient's face. Sometimes we need to further sculpt the implants by hand to make everything balance.

- The implant is inserted and sometimes stitched to more-solid internal facial features.

- The incision is then closed, often with one stitch.

The procedure usually takes forty-five to ninety minutes. Sometimes it is performed in combination with forehead, eyelid, facelift, nasal, or chin surgery. When the most common implant, solid silicone, is used, supportive tissue eventually forms around the implant after a few weeks. It is important to note that unlike breast implants that are made of liquid silicone and can rupture, cheek implants are solid and safer. Once fully healed, the implant feels like your normal underlying bone structure.

Reducing Chipmunk Cheeks: Buccal Fat Removal

Sometimes the cheeks can be too full and round in the lower aspect of the face, often described by patients as "chipmunk cheeks." We learned in chapter 2 that in beautiful faces, the upper cheeks should be 1.618 times wider than the lower face—the Golden Proportion. In chipmunk cheeks, the upper and lower cheeks are equal in width or a 1 to 1 ratio, which is not ideal or as attractive.

To create beautiful cheeks in this situation, a cheek-reduction technique called a buccal fat pad removal can be performed. The buccal fat pad is located at the bottom of the cheeks on either side of the corner of the mouth. Removal of these fat pads can slim the lower face, creating the appearance of higher cheekbones. After this surgery the ratio of the upper cheeks to the lower face goes from being 1 to 1 to closer to the Golden Ratio of beauty of 1.618 to 1.

During buccal fat pad removal an incision is made inside the mouth, about a half inch in length opposite the upper molar teeth. As much of the fat pad is removed as is necessary to achieve the desired contour. Removing the entire fat pad, however, is not suggested because it can create a hollowed face. As we get older and lose facial volume, the cheek can sink more, so this operation must be executed with artistry and precision.

Chin Contouring

In many instances, the face may require a chin augmentation to harmonize the features of the face. Interestingly, chin augmentation can improve the appearance of the nose, making it look smaller. A chin that is weak will make a larger nose the pinnacle of the face and draw attention to it. An appropriately sized chin after an augmentation

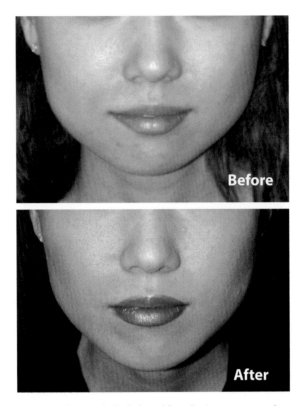

Figure 31. Patient who had a buccal fat reduction surgery to reduce "chipmunk cheeks" and bring more highlights to the cheek bones. She also had chin augmentation at the same time.

will balance the lower face with the midsection of the face, drawing attention away from a larger nose. Chin augmentation will also reduce the appearance of early jowling along the neck and jawline, creating a mini-facelift appearance. As such, it sometimes is combined with liposuction under the neck to create a neck-lift appearance, as described in chapter 12.

When performing chin augmentation, less is more. An overly strong chin can look masculine in a woman and like Abe Lincoln in a man. As a general rule, a woman's chin should ideally be located just behind a line drawn vertically down from where the nose and upper lip meet. In men, it should be at this line or slightly in front of it. A stronger square chin and jawline is ideal in men. In women, a chin that is softer and comes to more of a point, although not pointy, is desirable. People are often afraid of chin augmentation surgery

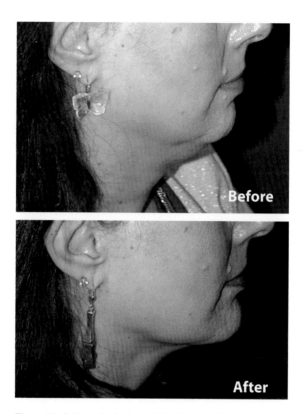

Figure 32. Patient who had a combination of a chin augmentation and a neck liposuction to create a tighter looking neck and jawline.

because many doctors use "button" chin implants, which come only in small, medium, and large and do not look natural because they exaggerate the area.

Chin implants come in hundreds of different shapes and sizes, so that the correct implant shape to harmonize with your cheeks and other facial features can be chosen. This is the artistry of plastic surgery.

Chin augmentation surgery is performed through a small incision inside the lower lip between it and the gums or in the natural crease line just underneath the chin. The overlying tissues are lifted off the chin bone, creating a space where an implant can be placed over the deficient bone of the skeleton. Fine sutures are used to close the incisions, and the scar is usually imperceptible.

Even though I perform this procedure with both approaches, I prefer the incision under the chin. When the implants are placed through an incision inside the mouth, a ligament that holds the lip to the chin gets cut, which can result in a subtle change in the appearance of the lower lip in a small percentage of cases.

Additionally, it has been shown in studies that, with the approach from inside the mouth, the implants can shift in a higher percentage of cases. I educate my patients about the pros and cons and allow them to make the final decision. If an implant twists, it requires revision surgery and screwing of the implant to the jawbone to correct the problem.

Men who have a narrow width to the outer aspects of their jaw by their ears but want an even stronger jawline are candidates for jawline implants. This is not a common procedure in women as the jawline should be balanced and defined but softer and more understated. Jawline implant procedures are different from those of chin implants and are performed along with chin augmentation.

Jaw implants are also referred to as gonial angle implants because they augment the angle of the jaw (the gonial angle). While this is common for people with small jaws, it also brings more masculinity and balance to the male face. These implants are generally placed through incisions inside the mouth, farther back along the jawline, at the crease where the inside of your lower lips and gums meet. The material most commonly used in jaw implants is a material called Medpor which your body grows into. It is more stable than silicone. Jaw implants need to be harder and more stable as the chewing muscles push against them. For this reason, they are usually screwed in position.

One other procedure in chin reshaping is chin reduction surgery. Although it is also performed in men, this is most common used with women who have a stronger jawline than desired, which gives their face a harder, more masculine appearance. The approach uses the same incisions as used in chin implantation discussed above, and the size of the bone is reduced by filing or burring it down.

References

Binder, W.J., B. Azizzadeh. 2008. Malar and submalar augmentation. *Facial Plastic Surgery Clinics of North America.* Feb; 16(1): 11-32.

Matarasso, A. 2006. Managing the buccal fat pad. *Aesthetic Surgery Journal.* May-Jun; 26(3): 330-336.

Yaremchuk, M.J. 2003. Improving aesthetic outcomes after alloplastic chin augmentation. *Plastic Reconstructive Surgery.* Oct; 112(5): 1422-1432; discussion 1433-1434.

14 Lip Augmentation

According to the American Academy of Facial and Reconstructive Surgery, lip augmentation using injectable fillers was one of the most common facial plastic procedures performed in 2011. In fact, the number of people having lip augmentation increased more than the number receiving any other facial procedure.

There are two major types of lip augmentation. Nonsurgical lip augmentation is accomplished by injecting fillers, whether temporary, permanent, or your own body's fat. Further information on the types of fillers available and their advantages and disadvantages are discussed in chapters 4, 5, and 6. The other type of augmentation is a surgical treatment, and there are many different types of lip augmentation surgery, which I will discuss later.

Beautiful lips also respect the Golden Ratio. As described in chapter 2, the lower lip should be larger than the upper lip, or, according to this Golden Proportion, the lower lip should be 1.618 times larger than the upper lip. The distance from the points of the upper lip, called the peaks of Cupid's bow, to the corner of the mouth should be 1.618 times the distance between the points of the center of the lip. A diagram (figure 7) of these proportions can be seen in chapter 2.

As we age, our lips lose their fullness, which makes them appear older. Lip skin is very thin and lips have no oil glands, which is why they dry out and chap. Lips descend because of loss of support. The distance between the tip of the nose and the upper lip gets longer over time as well. Sometimes the upper lip becomes so long that it hangs over the upper teeth, and the face can take on an almost apelike appearance.

Full lips are becoming increasingly desirable because they connote youth, beauty, and sex appeal. Think Angelina Jolie and Scarlett

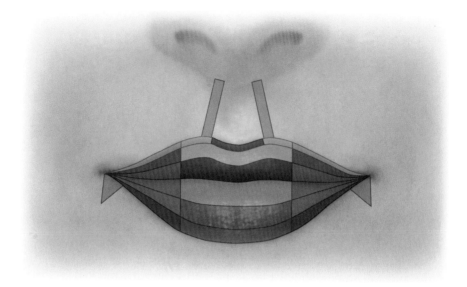

Figure 33. Illustration demonstrating fifteen different anatomic zones used to direct lip augmentation with injectable fillers. These zones are injected differentially to create natural appearing customized lips, while avoiding an overfilled "trout pout" look.

Johansson. Your lips are an essential component of facial symmetry and aesthetics. Anthropometric studies have shown that wider and fuller lips in relation to facial width, as well as a more defined Cupid's bow, are a mark of female attractiveness. Lip shrinkage disrupts facial harmony and can result in the perception that your nasal tip or jawline is too large for your face.

Many of my patients are afraid of having lip augmentation, since they don't want a "trout pout" or "duck lips." Examples of these kinds of lips are seen in celebs like Meg Ryan, Donatella Versace, Melanie

> A great lip augmentation and rejuvenation addresses all of these areas: the visible portion of the lip (the vermillion), the outer mouth (laugh lines), the edges of the lips (lipstick lines), and the inner lip.

Griffith, and Lisa Rinna, for starters. In an ideal situation, even if one has full, beautiful lips, the upper lip should be smaller than the lower lip as described above for the Golden Proportion. In the celebrity cases just mentioned, that proportion becomes reversed with the upper lip being too big and "ducky." As the upper lip becomes overfilled, the

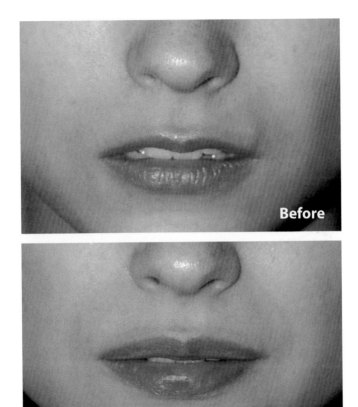

Figure 34. This patient had a V to Y lip augmentation, rolling the lips from the inside out to create fuller lips.

peaks of the natural Cupid's bow are also lost, resulting in an unnatural lip that goes straight across and looks like a filled sausage.

Nonsurgical Lip Augmentation

The traditional lip augmentation technique currently favored by plastic surgeons and dermatologists worldwide involves injecting a filler into the lip border, which can make the lip look unnatural and overstuffed. I have developed a classification system for the placement of injectable fillers during lip augmentation that targets fifteen different anatomic zones, instead of injecting only the lip-line site (vermillion border), to deliver beautiful and pouty lips that look completely natural.

Every person's lips are imbalanced in different ways, so we inject different zones on essentially every person to establish the Golden

121

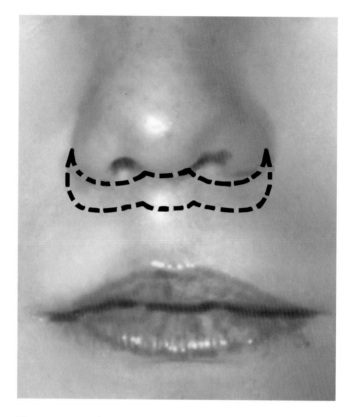

Figure 35. Incision for a "Bull's Horn" lip lift is hidden underneath the nose.

Proportion described above. In some patients we may inject only three zones, and, in another, ten zones to attain the correct size and proportional shape. Lipstick bleed lines and a downturned mouth can also be corrected at the same time, as described in chapter 4's section on temporary and permanent facial fillers. Fat transfer can also be used. This procedure is performed by suctioning fat from the abdomen or thighs and transferring the fat with specialized syringes and instruments to the area to be treated. These results can last up to two years in most cases, and a touch-up can be done at any time to maintain the desired volume. While most lip injections are temporary, silicone injections can yield permanent results.

Surgical Lip Augmentation

For people with naturally thin lips who are seeking a more permanent solution and do not want silicone in their lips, I can also perform more invasive procedures that will require a week or two of recovery. The procedures I perform include a technique called V-to-Y lip augmentation and lip lifting. The V-to-Y lip advancement surgery procedure delivers permanent, voluptuous lips like Angelina Jolie's. This technique uses small imperceptible incisions on the inside of the lips. The lip is rolled out from the inside out, making it pouty and full. Because the incisions are on the inside of the lips, there are no visible scars. The results of this procedure are permanent.

I performed studies on this technique, and it can be adjusted so that lips are augmented more subtly or more aggressively (as in cases with very thin lips). The upper and lower lips can be augmented differentially so that the Golden Proportion can be attained. Also, this operation increases the curvature of Cupid's bow, which can improve the Golden Ratio of the upper lip. The downside to this operation is a longer-than-usual recovery time of four to six weeks during which the lips will look swollen.

There are new lip implants, similar to the encased liquid silicone implants used for breast augmentation, that are surgically inserted into the lips. I do not suggest solid plastic implants like these to my patients

Ask for only temporary filler products for the lips that have a good safety record and have been on the market for many years, not just a few months. Restylane is the only filler in the United States to receive FDA approval for lips.

because they have a small but significant rate of extruding through the skin, causing scarring. The reason for this is our lips are soft and move a lot, so over time a more solid implant can force its way out of the body.

The lip-lift procedure targets only the upper lip, elevating it to reveal a broader smile. This procedure exposes more of the upper teeth at rest that tend to be covered as we age. It increases the volume of the upper lip, and for those with a very thin upper lip it can bring it into a better aesthetic proportion with the lower lip. Additionally, this procedure can be executed to elevate different sections of the lip along the central Cupid's bow. The result is that a Golden Ratio can be created between the Cupid's bow apexes that are not present in a flat lip. One popular type of upper-lip lift is called the Bull's Horn Lip Lift. During this procedure, an incision is made just beneath your nose. A tiny strip of skin and tissue is removed, and the upper lip is raised to its new position. With this lip lift, your scar is virtually undetectable. The procedure takes about forty-five minutes and recovery time is about five to seven days.

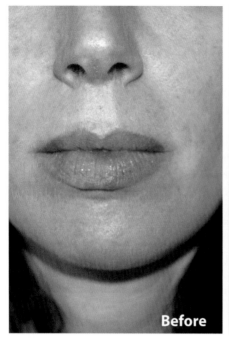
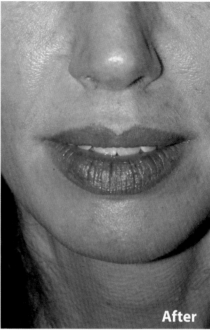

Figure 36. Patient who had a "Bull's Horn" lip lift. The distance between the upper lip and nose is shortened, the lip appears fuller, and the upper teeth can now be seen, which is aesthetically more pleasing.

Other upper lip lift procedures vary, based on where the incision is placed. For example, a Gull Wing Lift removes a strip of skin above the border of your upper lip. The cutout is M-shaped to advance the border of your upper lip. The incision is made where the pink part of your upper lip meets the skin under the nose. This lip lift leaves a visible scar and, as a result, is not as desirable as other techniques.

References

Austin, H. 1986. The lip lift. *Plastic and Reconstructive Surgery.* 77: 990.

Jacono, A.A. 2008. A new classification of lip zones to customize injectable lip augmentation. *Archives of Facial Plastic Surgery.* Jan-Feb; 10(1): 25-29.

Jacono, A.A., V.C. Quatela. 2004. Quantitative analysis of lip appearance after V-Y lip augmentation. *Archives of Facial Plastic Surgery.* May-Jun; 6(3): 172-177.

15 The Art of Rhinoplasty

The definition of rhinoplasty is shaping the nose. It is more commonly referred to as a "nose job." Every year more than half a million people will consult a facial plastic surgeon to improve the appearance of their nose. Because the nose is the most defining characteristic of the face, even a slight alteration can greatly improve one's appearance. For example, when there is a large hump on the nose in profile, the excess bone and cartilage can be removed, resulting in a straighter and flatter appearance.

Evaluating Your Nose

I always favor creating a natural rhinoplasty result, one that is aesthetically balanced to the face. I do not think that using established proportions of beauty is acceptable regarding the nose. Patients have very specific ideas about how they want their nose to look, and some of these desires do not respect Golden Proportions. For example, some patients may want to maintain some part of a nose hump to maintain some of their identity whereas others may want a straight bridge.

Further, some ethnicities have unique nasal characteristics. For people who want a nose job, it is typical for all races to want a change of appearance in their nose without diminishing their cultural background or heritage. Opinions are so diverse among different people about the ideal nose shape that it is similar to differing preferences about something as simple as color in clothing. That is why I use digital photography and computer imaging software to simulate how patients will look after surgery. Digital morphing is crucial to help define how patients want their nose to look. I do not give everyone the same nose, and I customize the surgery to enhance each individual's

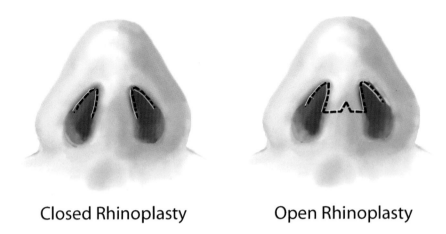

Closed Rhinoplasty   Open Rhinoplasty

Figure 37. Incisions for closed and open rhinoplasty. The closed approach has only internal incisions inside the nostrils. The external approach has a small incision that connects the two internal nostril incisions; this provides exposure to the nasal tip allowing for more nasal tip reshaping.

unique aesthetic balance. This approach becomes the road map for surgery. There needs to be a merging of good techniques, aesthetic understanding by the surgeon, and the desire of the patient as defined by digital morphing to prevent unwanted results.

Rhinoplasty: Open or Closed?

Rhinoplasty can be performed through an open or closed approach, with the closed approach having all internal incisions that are not visible, and the open approach requiring a well-hidden, tiny incision across the base of the nose. Some surgeons only perform open rhinoplasty and some perform only closed. I perform both open and closed rhinoplasty, choosing the best approach depending upon the goals of the surgery. There are some modifications of the nose, especially some nasal tip maneuvers, that can be executed only through an open rhinoplasty approach. Additionally, revision rhinoplasty surgery is often best performed through an open approach as it allows the surgeon more access to deal with scar tissue and cartilage distorted by prior surgery.

Reshaping Nose Cartilage

More sophisticated rhinoplasty surgeons will reshape the cartilages of the tip of the nose rather than cut away the supportive structure of the nasal tip. Cutting away the cartilage will destabilize the nose and

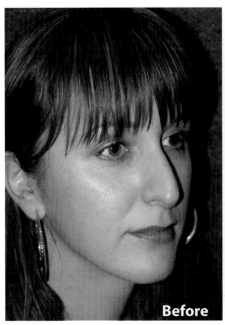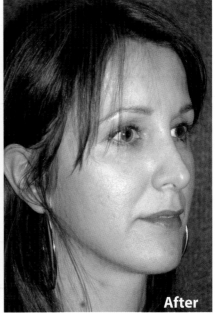

Before   **After**

Figure 38. Patient who had open rhinoplasty. Notice reduction of the nasal bridge hump as well as lifting and refining of the tip. The nose looks natural.

make it more likely to collapse and have problems. Also, sculpting the nasal bones of the bridge by shaving, rather than breaking, the nose is a new technique that will dramatically decrease recovery time after surgery. Breaking the bones causes bruises around the eyes, which can take a few weeks to resolve.

Some patients require augmentation rhinoplasty where cartilage grafting is required. Others have had prior rhinoplasty that requires a revision that also may need structure added back to the nose with cartilage grafting. This cartilage can be obtained from inside the nose, from the ear, and, in severe multiple revision cases, from the ribs. Skull bone called calvarial bone may be required in the worst of cases. Whenever tissue is transplanted to the nose, recoveries are longer as the body has to grow into them.

Ethnic Rhinoplasty

Common techniques used in ethnic rhinoplasty include augmentation (building up) of a flat nasal bridge, lengthening and refining a wide and short nasal tip, and narrowing the base of the nostrils. This is different from techniques used for Caucasian noses where rhino-

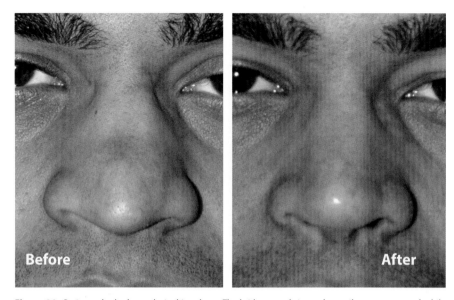

Figure 39. Patient who had an ethnic rhinoplasty. The bridge, nasal tip, and nostrils were narrowed while maintaining natural proportion and "heritage" of the nose.

plasty often removes cartilage and bone because the nose is too long, too big, or overprojected. Ethnic nose job techniques can be used to improve the appearance of African-American, Hispanic, Middle Eastern, and Asian noses, while respecting and maintaining the patient's ethnic heritage. To build up the nose in rhinoplasty surgery, I prefer to use your body's natural cartilage (as noted above) instead of implants (such as silicone, Gore-Tex, or Medpore), since foreign substances have a tendency to become infected or are pushed out of the nose (extruded) over the years following surgery.

When narrowing the nostrils during ethnic rhinoplasty surgery, it is necessary to remove extra skin from the nostrils by making an incision in the crease of the nostril where it meets the cheek. This procedure is called an alar base reduction. Because the incision is well hidden, the incision lines heal well and are not noticeable.

When interviewing a doctor for surgery during a consultation, you should be allowed to see hundreds of examples of their work. During your review of these photos, make sure that all the noses do not look the same because that indicates that the doctor has a "cookie-cutter" approach to surgery and your nose will look just like all the others.

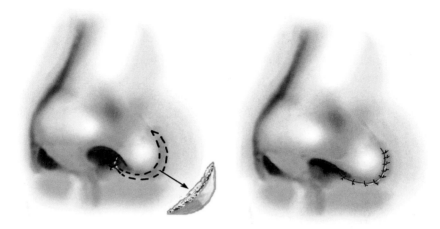

Figure 40. Illustration of the incisions for a nostril reduction surgery, which is called an alar base reduction. The incision is well hidden in the natural groove between the nose and cheek.

Revision Rhinoplasty

The unfortunate truth about rhinoplasty is that somewhere between 10 and 20 percent of surgeries performed in the United States require revision surgery either because the person undergoing the surgery is not satisfied with its look or because of postsurgery breathing problems.

Many times, revision rhinoplasty requires a nose to be reduced in size. Common problems include a nasal hump being left behind (bump on the bridge towards the tip called a pollybeak deformity because it makes the nose look like the beak of a bird), a tip remains wide and lacks definition, a tip is still droopy, or the nostrils are too wide.

Because the problems are different for each patient, the revision rhinoplasty surgery needs to be customized to each individual's unique problems. The maneuvers necessary may be as simple as removing some more cartilage or bone or reshaping the cartilages of the nose. If too much cartilage is removed from an overly aggressive nose job, the nose will collapse.

Performing cartilage grafting is necessary when the results of a rhinoplasty give an unnatural "pinched tip," "pig nose," or collapsed middle bridge called an inverted V deformity. The inverted V deformity is so-called because it looks like someone drew an upside-down letter "V" in the middle of the nose.

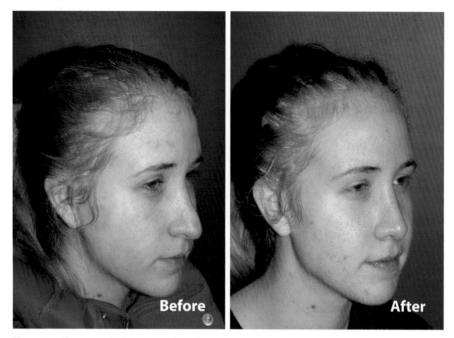

Figure 41. This patient had a revision rhinoplasty. Her prior surgery reduced a nasal hump but left the tip droopy and bulbous. Her revision surgery lifted the nasal tip, shortened the nose, and created a defined nasal tip that appears natural.

The best place to obtain cartilage in revision surgery is from nasal septum (a piece of cartilage inside the nose). When it is not available due to prior surgery, cartilage from behind the ears or the ribs can be used. Cartilage is removed from the area around the ear canal through an incision that is often hidden behind the ear. The shape of the ear does not change. When cartilage is taken from the rib cage, a small incision about 1½ inches long is hidden underneath the breast in the crease or, in a man, at the bottom of the pectoralis muscle. In the most severe cases, calvarial bone from the skull can be harvested and used to restructure a completely collapsed nose called a "saddle nose." The incision for harvesting the bone is hidden in the hair.

A collapsed nose or collapsed middle bridge can create functional breathing issues. Fixing the aesthetic issues of the nose, which requires using cartilage to support the collapsed structures, can reverse breathing problems.

Revision rhinoplasty requires the expertise of a facial plastic and reconstructive surgeon who specializes in both revision cosmetic surgery and reconstructive surgery. I discuss how to find these doctors in chapter 17.

References

Mehta, U., K. Mazhar, A.S. Frankel. 2010. Accuracy of preoperative computer imaging in rhinoplasty. *Archives of Facial Plastic Surgery.* Nov-Dec; 12(6): 394-398.

Quatela, V.C., A.A. Jacono. Structural grafting in rhinoplasty. *Facial Plastic Surgery.* Nov; 18(4): 223-232.

Rohrich, R.J., K. Bolden. 2010. Ethnic rhinoplasty. *Clinical Plastic Surgery.* Apr; 37(2): 353-370.

Tebbetts, J.B. 2006. Open and closed rhinoplasty (minus the "versus"): Analyzing processes. *Aesthetic Surgery Journal.* Jul-Aug; 26(4): 456-459.

16 Men and Plastic Surgery

With the American male grooming market now worth $3.5 billion, men seem to be changing their attitude about a number of issues that seemed previously to be the preserve of women. Feeling the need to look youthful and appear dynamic well into their forties, fifties, sixties, and beyond has led to men rethinking their attitudes to pills, diet, exercise, face-care products, and cosmetic (plastic) surgery.

Men increasingly want to change the things they don't like to see in the mirror. Statistics available from the American Society of Aesthetic Plastic Surgery show that surgery is becoming increasingly popular with men as a way to deal with image maintenance and change.

- 84 percent of men surveyed believed that physical attractiveness contributed to success and power on the job.

- 42 percent felt that improving one thing about their face would help their career.

- 32 percent agreed that a more youthful appearance would positively impact job success.

The message is that the way you look can have a substantial impact on how you feel, your job, and your career. Today's economy and competitive job market is the overwhelming reason why interest in facial plastic surgery among men has risen so sharply in the past decade. Not only must one be qualified for a job, one must project a confident, youthful, and energetic look.

According to the American Academy of Facial Plastic and Reconstructive Surgeons, the most common surgeries performed on

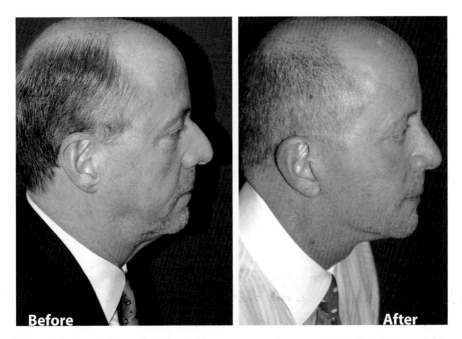

Figure 42. This man had rhinoplasty. The nasal hump was removed but a strong bridge that appears masculine was created. At the same time, he also had a lower eyelid lift with fat transposition and a facelift.

men were rhinoplasties, followed by hair transplants, blepharoplasty (eyelid-lift surgery), and finally neck-lift surgery. In male plastic surgery, the procedures are performed differently from in females in order to maintain a natural appearance that is not feminized. These details are important because men want to look like themselves, simply rejuvenated.

Rhinoplasty

Rhinoplasty in men is different from in women. Male noses have thicker skin and stronger bones and the aesthetic ideals in men are different. Male rhinoplasty has to address the thick skin in the nose to achieve excellent results. Also, removing the bump or lifting the tip has to be done very conservatively, in order not to feminize the appearance of the nose. A small upturned nose on a man looks out of place. Additionally, the nose has to fit other facial features of the male face to achieve a natural outcome. The angle between nose and upper lip in a male nose should not exceed 90 degrees, otherwise the nose appears too rotated or feminine. In the female nose, it should be 105 degrees or higher, depending on the distance between nose and lips and other features.

133

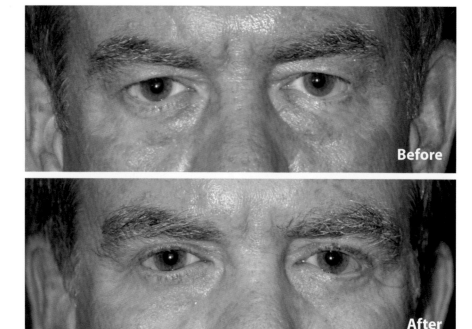

Figure 43. Patient who underwent upper and lower eyelid lifts. Notice how he looks refreshed yet masculine even though the brows are slightly heavy. A heavier brow is attractive in men. Browlifts often create a feminized appearance and should be avoided in men.

Hair Transplants

Hair transplants have changed since years past where men had obvious-looking "hair plugs." Today we transplant follicular unit micrografts. When performed by an experienced doctor, this technique results in hairlines that both look and function naturally, with minimal interference in lifestyle. Hair grafting has been performed for more than thirty years, but it is only in the past five years that technological advancements, as well as a greater appreciation of hairline aesthetics, have truly made the results of this procedure virtually undetectable. Hairs are taken from the back of the head from areas that are not susceptible to ever going bald, and transplanted into bald or thinning areas on the top and front of the head; this way, a permanent and natural-appearing full head of hair can be attained using the individual's own hairs. I discuss this in great detail in chapter 8.

Each follicular unit micrograft contains one, two, three, or occasionally four hairs. Usually a combination of these different-sized

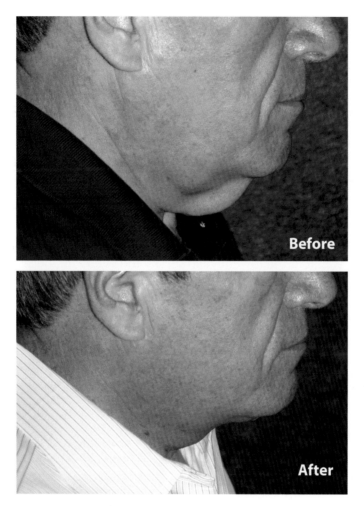

Figure 44. Patient is shown after a direct neck lift. The incision was placed under the chin. The healing time is half that of a traditional neck lift that has incisions behind the ears.

grafts is used in the hair restoration, with the one-hair grafts going up front in an irregular pattern along the hairline, and the two-, three-, and four-hair grafts placed farther behind to create more density. To attain the most natural result, each graft contains a single follicular unit, the collection of usually two to three hairs all within a tiny bunch, which is the way that hair grows naturally in most individuals.

By transplanting follicular units, the way hair grows naturally, the results of a hair transplantation are virtually undetectable. Precise planting of the transplants in a random pattern results in a natural-looking hairline that does not look like a telltale straight line. Follicular unit grafting is the most advanced procedure, requiring a team of trained assistants to cut each graft under the microscope.

Eyelid Lifts

In eyelid surgery for men, it is important not to change the shape of the eye. In women we usually like to re-create the almond eyelid shape of youth. In men, we make an incision inside the eyelids, so no scar is created and the shape of the eye is maintained. Additionally, the lower eyelid bags that make us look tired are repositioned into the deep under eyelid circles, making the eyelids look rejuvenated, not tired. It is not uncommon for men to hear "You look tired and overworked" because of their eyelid appearance. It is important to preserve the fat of the lower eyelid during the eyelid lift, because if the fat bags are removed, it makes the eyes look sunken and potentially sickly.

Avoiding Brow Lifts for Men

As I stated in earlier, I do not suggest brow-lift surgery for the vast majority of men as they age. I think the reasons set forth earlier are worth repeating. When we look at the brow position of iconic leading men in Hollywood who are considered to be very attractive, like Brad Pitt and Tom Cruise, we notice that they have heavy brows. A heavier brow accentuates the bridge of bone in the forehead right above the eyes that doctors call the supraorbital ridge, which is a male facial skeletal characteristic.

As mentioned earlier, since this ridge is accentuated with age, it is one of the reasons that men are said to become more handsome and distinguished as they get older. Additionally, brow orientation in men should go straight across this part of the forehead as it also accentuates this bony ridge, and not arch up above it (a feminine characteristic) as discussed above.

Neck Lifts

Men are as sensitive about their "turkey neck" as women are but do not usually want a facelift or neck-lift procedure. These procedures have longer recovery times and require more surgery. In men there is a procedure called a "direct neck skin excision" where we can make an incision under the chin and remove the hanging neck skin while tightening the neck muscles called platysma that sag with age. The immediate effect is that the jawline looks more defined, and it appears that the individual has lost weight because the heaviness under the neck has been removed. A more athletic and energetic appearance is the result. Because of men's bearded skin, the incision on the neck heals well and is camouflaged.

I have performed many surgeries like this on men in the financial industries who have taken only four or five days off from work for the procedure, which is easy to schedule in a busy work life. A small bandage can be placed over the area, and, if anyone asks what happened, simply say you had a cyst removed from your neck.

17 Choosing a Facial Plastic Surgeon

Where do you begin when looking for a qualified facial plastic surgeon? Facial cosmetic surgery has become extremely popular due to the competitiveness of today's society; everyone wants to look young and vibrant. Although it seems that everyone is having something "done," not many are so willing to announce it, let alone refer you to their doctor. Ideally, referrals are a great way for one to inspect a surgeon's work but are sometimes difficult to come by. So now what? Well, it's time to do some homework.

Surgeon Training and Certification

First, contact one of the boards listed below for recommendations or to check that the surgeon you are considering is board-certified. Not all cosmetic surgeons have the same training or certifications. Currently, there are five legitimate boards that are either a member board of the American Board of Medical Specialties (ABMS) or ABMS-equivalent boards. These boards include: the American Board of Facial Plastic and Reconstructive Surgery, the American Board of Plastic Surgery, the American Board of Dermatology, the American Board of Otolaryngology/Head and Neck Surgery, and the American Board of Ophthalmology.

The American Board of Facial Plastic and Reconstructive Surgery certifies surgeons in the specific specialty area of plastic surgery of the face. The only surgeons who even qualify to take this specialists' board exam are either board-certified diplomates of the American Board of Otolaryngology/Head and Neck Surgery, or of the American Board of Plastic Surgery. The American Medical Association (AMA) recognizes the American Board of Otolaryngology/Head and Neck Surgery, the

American Board of Plastic Surgery, and the American Board of Facial Plastic and Reconstructive Surgery as legitimate certifying boards to test the qualifications of surgeons to perform facial plastic surgery.

Board-certified and fellowship-trained facial plastic surgeons complete five years of a otolaryngology/head and neck surgery residency during which they operate only on the face, nose, eyelids, head, and neck. During this time, they perform cancer surgery for the head and neck, nose, and face, including reconstructive surgery on the face. They also perform cosmetic procedures, such as rhinoplasty, eyelid lifting, and facelifting during this time. They then go on to complete an additional year of fellowship training specializing further in the most updated techniques in facial plastic and reconstructive surgery. This fellowship is sponsored by the American Academy of Facial Plastic and Reconstructive Surgery.

Confirming that a surgeon has board certification is just the beginning. Once you have discovered that the surgeon has the appropriate boards, it is time to look at before-and-after photographs of some of their patients. Browse through their online photo gallery. A skilled surgeon should have many before-and-after photographs on their site. It is also important to note whether you like the surgeon's aesthetic. Cosmetic surgery is both a skill and an art; just because a doctor has all the required credentials doesn't necessarily mean that he or she is able to create the look you desire.

You should also check your doctor's hospital affiliations. If a physician has privileges to perform surgery at an accredited hospital, this demonstrates that his or her performance and credentials are subject to regular scrutiny. While most plastic surgeons perform surgery only in their office, they do have privileges to perform surgery at a local hospital. If a doctor does not have these privileges, do not use that doctor.

Scheduling a Consultation

Your next step is to schedule a consultation. Understand that if you choose to have surgery with this doctor, you will be spending quite a bit of time in the office, so it is important that you feel comfortable there. A good doctor will listen to your concerns, answer all your questions, and explain all risks and benefits of the procedures you are interested in. Some surgeons use digital morphing programs to simulate the changes you may expect from having facial cosmetic surgery. Many have found this to be a helpful tool.

After meeting with the surgeon, it is most likely you will meet with a patient care coordinator who will discuss financing, book your surgery dates, give you pre- and postoperative instructions, and answer any other questions you may have. If you would like to speak with a patient who has undergone the same procedure you are considering, the patient care coordinator can put you in touch with one. Skilled surgeons usually have happy patients who are willing to share their experiences with someone planning to have a similar procedure.

Remember, you can't hide your face, so the decision to have facial plastic surgery will be one of the most important decisions you will make. If you still have further questions, you may wish to have a second consultation with your surgeon.

18 Pro-Bono Surgery: You Can Help

As a facial plastic and reconstructive surgeon, I've long been grateful to specialize in a field where I can offer my skills and services to the benefit of others. In my profession, you speak to a very basic human need to be confident in one's appearance. From working with aesthetic patients looking for a confidence boost in their marriage or career, to the domestic-violence victim, cancer patient, or accident victim looking to rebuild his or her life, I have found that it is both rewarding and impactful to satisfy a patient's need to feel whole and confident in the face they're showing the world.

Face to Face: The Domestic-Violence Project

Early in my career, I was deeply moved by a patient who was the tragic victim of domestic violence. This was a female patient who returned with a shattered nose months after I performed reconstructive rhinoplasty on her twisted nose. It turns out it was her husband, not a car accident, that was responsible for her defacement. She inspired me to rally around this silent epidemic and put forth my medical skills to improve the lives of those affected. It was at this point I became involved in Face to Face: The National Domestic Violence project (www.facetofacesurgery.org). This program was started by the American Academy of Facial Plastic and Reconstructive Surgery (AAFPRS) and the National Coalition Against Domestic Violence and offers complimentary consultations, surgery, counseling, and support to shattered victims of domestic abuse who otherwise would not be able to afford reconstructive or facial plastic surgery treatment. I have served as national chairman of the Face to Face Committee of the AAFPRS, and I am currently the senior advisor.

141

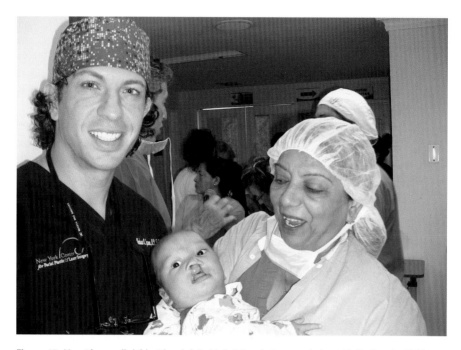

Figure 45. Me with a small child with a cleft lip birth defect during my mission with Healing the Children in Santa Marta, Colombia.

After a decade of involvement with this program, these patients have become like my extended family and give me a renewed energy that I bring to all of the patients in my practice. On the local level, my regular patients are also involved through an annual gala I hold to raise money on behalf of domestic violence victims in Long Island through the Nassau County Coalition Against Domestic Violence. Not only does this event raise awareness of this pervasive problem, but it also helps my aesthetic patients identify more with the core ideals of my practice.

Healing the Children

In addition to domestic violence awareness, I donate my time and services as a volunteer surgeon to Healing the Children (www.htcne. org) for the past five years. Healing the Children is an organization whose mission is to heal children with cleft lip and palates, birth defects, vascular tumors, burns, and other deformities and whose families don't have access to or cannot afford treatment. This kind of involvement means leaving my practice several times a year to travel

142

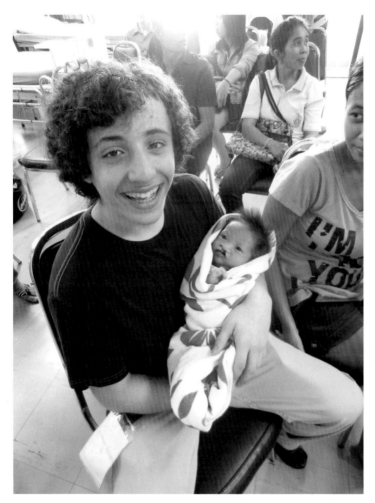

Figure 46. On his first mission with me in Thailand, my son, Andrew Jason Jacono, holds a five-week- old child with a cleft lip and palate deformity.

to third-world countries. I regularly travel to South America, Central America, and Southeast Asia where the rate of these birth defects is ten times what we see in the United States. It is unclear whether these statistics are related to environmental factors or genetics.

During an average visit of 10 days to a location, we screen 150 children and operate on about 75; unfortunately we cannot help every child when we go, so we must treat the youngest children first and come back the following year to these sites to perform surgery on those we couldn't get to previously. I cannot describe the joy I feel when I hand a nine-month-old child with a cleft lip back to his or her mother; the baby has gone into the operating room disfigured and come out one hour later with a normal and repaired face.

I was blessed to be able take my fourteen-year-old son to my last trip to Thailand as an ancillary staff member. One day about a year ago he told me he would like to come and help. I was surprised and proud at the same time and encouraged him to participate. It was

> Ten percent of the proceeds of this book will go to charitable causes. I am deeply committed to combating domestic violence and helping children born with cleft lip birth defects.

a life-transforming experience for both of us, and I look forward to traveling on future trips with him. He has a separate fund-raising effort for healing the children called T.H.A.I. (Through Healing All Indigent) Children Missions that raises money for Healing the Children. You can donate online at www.thaichildrenmissions.com.

If you want to get involved, please contact either of these two organizations by going to their websites as listed above. We always need volunteers to help and, of course, financial support so that we can continue this important work.

Index

About the Author

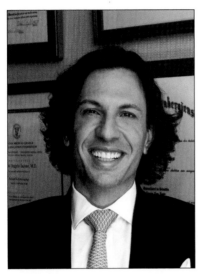

Andrew Jacono, M.D., F.A.C.S., is a dual board-certified facial plastic and reconstructive surgeon in Manhattan, specializing in minimally invasive facial rejuvenation. His extensive background in head and neck surgery and subspecialty training in facial plastic surgery give him a unique knowledge of the face and its underlying structures. Dr. Jacono is director of the New York Center for Facial Plastic & Laser Surgery and J SPA Medical Day Spa in Great Neck, New York. He is assistant clinical professor in the Facial Plastic and Reconstructive Surgery Division at the New York Eye and Ear Infirmary and Albert Einstein College of Medicine. He is section head of Facial Plastic Surgery at North Shore University Hospital and fellowship director for the American Academy of Facial Plastic and Reconstructive Surgery.

In addition to his aesthetic work, Dr. Jacono is the senior advisor to FACE TO FACE, a national project offering pro bono consultation and surgery to victims of domestic violence. Dr. Jacono's work with domestic violence victims has been chronicled in the television series *Facing Trauma* on the Oprah Winfrey Network and Discovery Fit & Health networks. *Facing Trauma* shares the stories of women who have been left disfigured from violent circumstances and follows Dr.

Jacono and his team as they work to heal both the internal and external scars of victims. He also volunteers for Healing the Children, which helps children throughout the world receive surgeries such as cleft lip and palate reconstruction, which would otherwise be unavailable to them due to a lack of medical and financial resources.

Dr. Jacono is a Castle Connolly top doctor and has been elected as one of America's top plastic surgeons by the Consumers Research Council of America and Super Doctors. He has been featured as one of New York City's leading plastic surgeons in *The New York Times*. His efforts were recognized by U.S. Congresswoman Carolyn McCarthy and the Center for the Women of New York for his contributions to women's welfare.

Dr. Jacono has lectured about cutting-edge facial plastic surgery techniques at conferences around the world. He has also published extensively in medical literature, including the *Aesthetic Surgery Journal* and *Archives of Facial Plastic Surgery*. His highly acclaimed first book was entitled *Face the Facts: The Truth About Facial Plastic Surgery Procedures That Do and Don't Work*. As a leading expert in his field, he has been featured on *Good Morning America, Anderson, CNBC*, and *CNN* and in *USA Today, Details, Parade, Huffington Post*, and *Newsweek*, among others.

Dr. Jacono currently performs surgery at the following hospitals:

- Lenox Hill Hospital, New York, NY
- The New York Eye and Ear Infirmary, New York, NY
- The Manhattan Eye, Ear and Throat Hospital, New York, NY
- North Shore University Hospital, Manhasset, NY
- Long Island Jewish Hospital, New Hyde Park, NY
- Saint Francis Hospital, Roslyn, NY
- Winthrop University Hospital, Mineola, NY

To learn more about Dr. Jacono and his practice, visit **www.newyorkfacialplasticsurgery.com.** You can also find him on Facebook (Andrew Jacono, MD-The New York Center for Facial Plastic and Laser Surgery) and Twitter (@drjacono).

Consumer Health Titles from Addicus Books

Visit our online catalog at www.AddicusBooks.com

To Order Books:
Visit us online at: www.AddicusBooks.com
Call toll free: (800) 352-2873

For discounts on bulk purchases, call our Special Sales Department at
(402) 330-7493.
Or email us at: info@AddicusBooks.com

Addicus Books
P. O. Box 45327
Omaha, NE 68145

Addicus Books is dedicated to publishing consumer health books that comfort and educate.